Table of Contents

Atkins Diet Recipe Book

Breakfasts

Smoothies

Lunches

Dinners

Side Dishes

Salads

Soups

Fat Bombs

Desserts

Atkins Diet Recipe Book

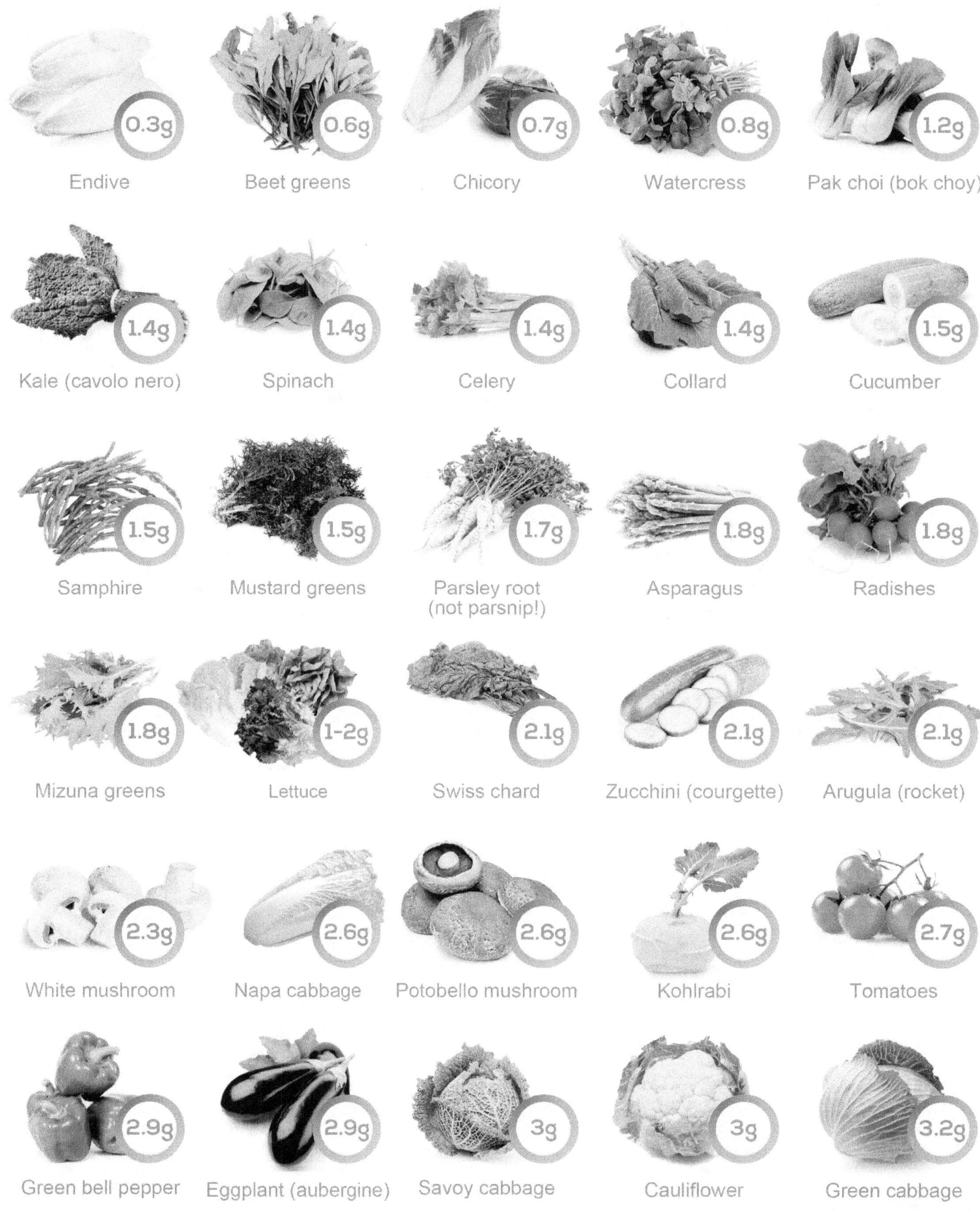

0.3g
Endive
0.6g
Beet greens
0.7g
Chicory
0.8g
Watercress
1.2g
Pak choi (bok choy)
1.4g
Kale (cavolo nero)
1.4g
Spinach
1.4g
Celery
1.4g
Collard
1.5g
Cucumber
1.5g
Samphire
1.5g
Mustard greens
1.7g
Parsley root
(not parsnip!)
1.8g
Asparagus
1.8g
Radishes
1.8g
Mizuna greens
1-2g
Lettuce
2.1g
Swiss chard
2.1g
Zucchini (courgette)
2.1g
Arugula (rocket)
2.3g
White mushroom
2.6g
Napa cabbage
2.6g
Potobello mushroom
2.6g
Kohlrabi
2.7g
Tomatoes
2.9g
Green bell pepper
2.9g
Eggplant (aubergine)
3g
Savoy cabbage
3g
Cauliflower
3.2g
Green cabbage
BEST
CARBS
WORST

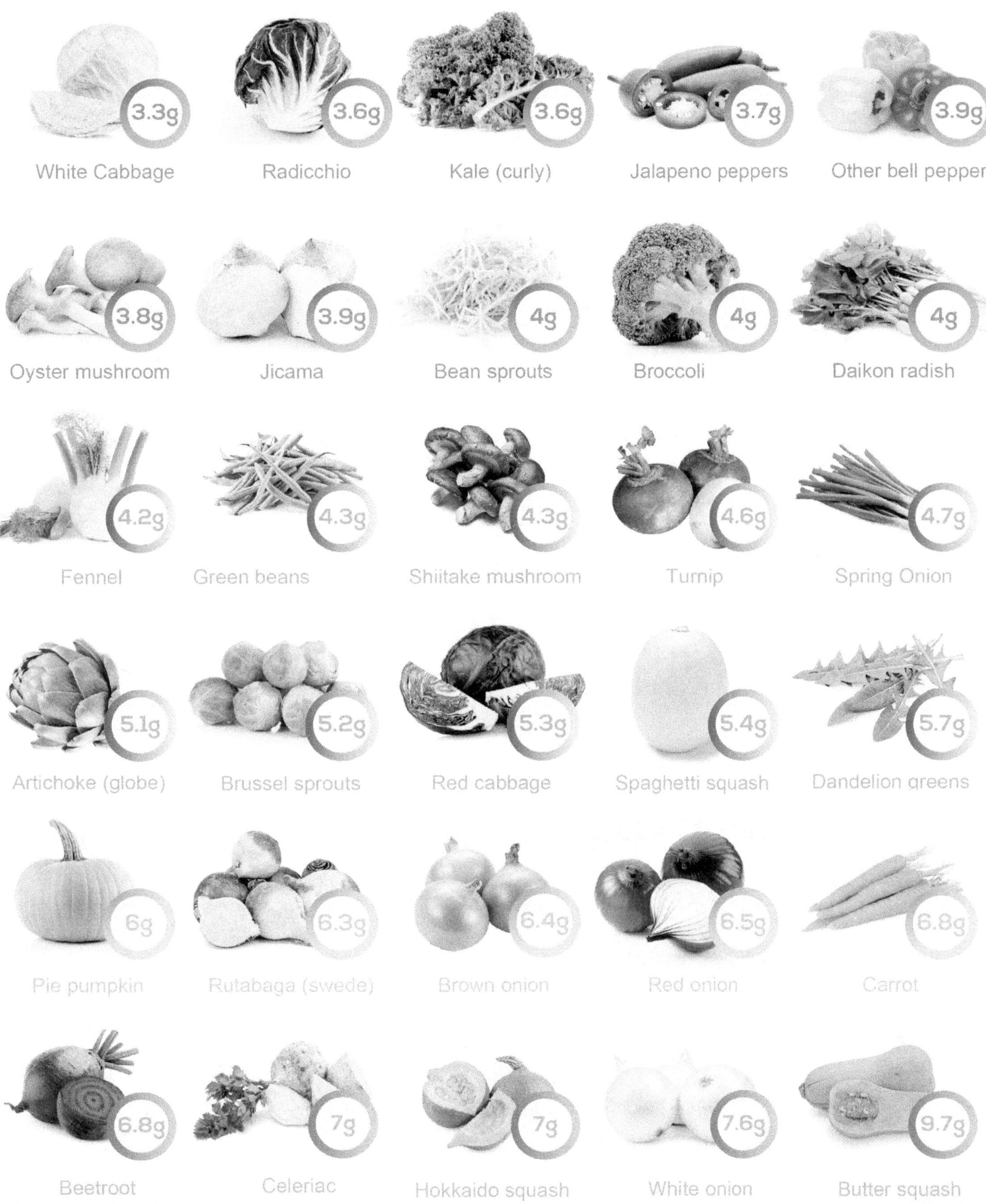

3.3g
White Cabbage
3.6g
Radicchio
3.6g
Kale (curly)
3.7g
Jalapeno peppers
3.9g
Other bell pepper
3.8g
Oyster mushroom
3.9g
Jicama
4g
Bean sprouts
4g
Broccoli
4g
Daikon radish
4.2g
Fennel
4.3g
Green beans
4.3g
Shiitake mushroom
4.6g
Turnip
4.7g
Spring Onion
5.1g
Artichoke (globe)
5.2g
Brussel sprouts
5.3g
Red cabbage
5.4g
Spaghetti squash
5.7g
Dandelion greens
6g
Pie pumpkin
6.3g
Rutabaga (swede)
6.4g
Brown onion
6.5g
Red onion
6.8g
Carrot
6.8g
Beetroot
7g
Celeriac
7g
Hokkaido squash
7.6g
White onion
9.7g
Butter squash
BEST
CARBS
WORST

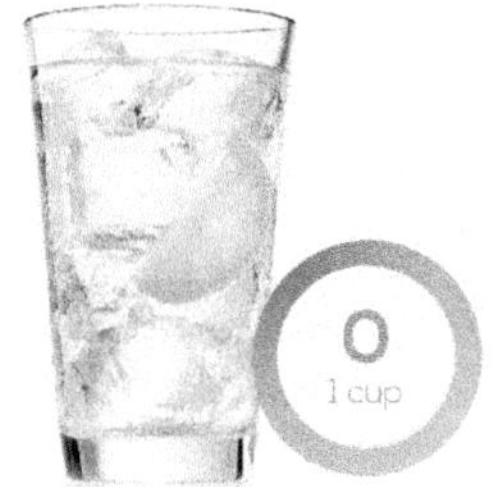

0
1 cup

Water with lemon

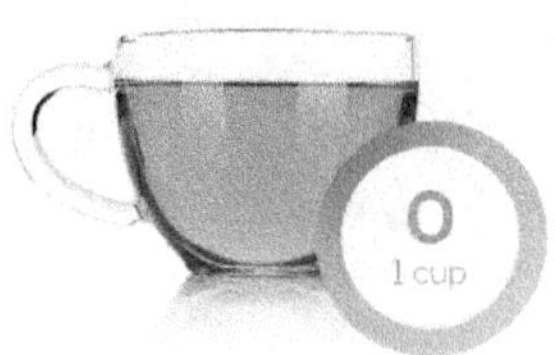

0
1 cup

Tea

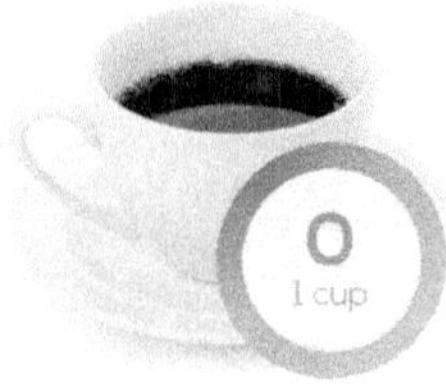

0
1 cup

Coffee

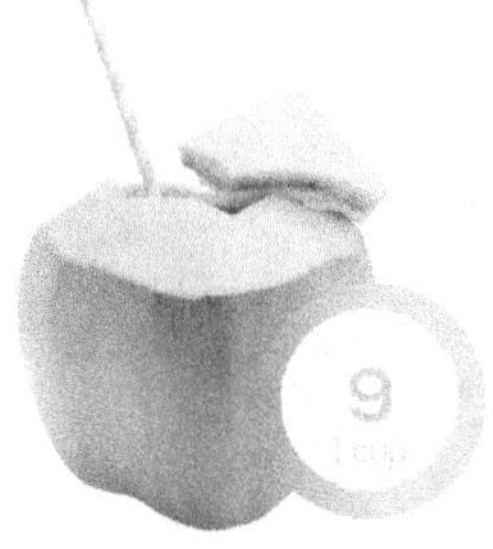

9
1 cup

Coconut water

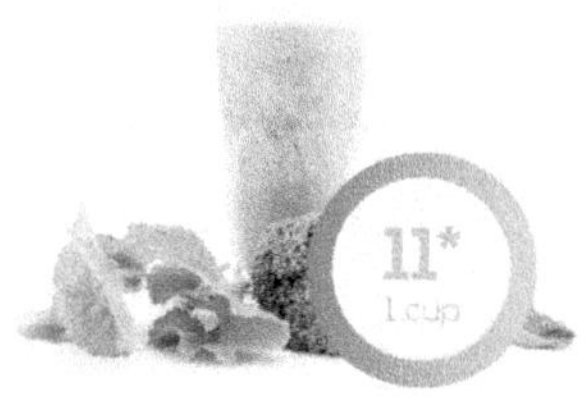

11*
1 cup

Vegetable juice

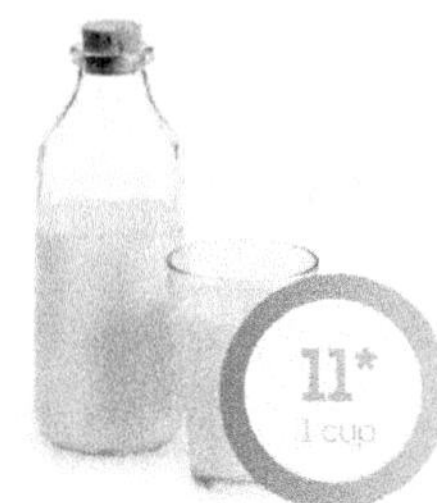

11*
1 cup

Milk

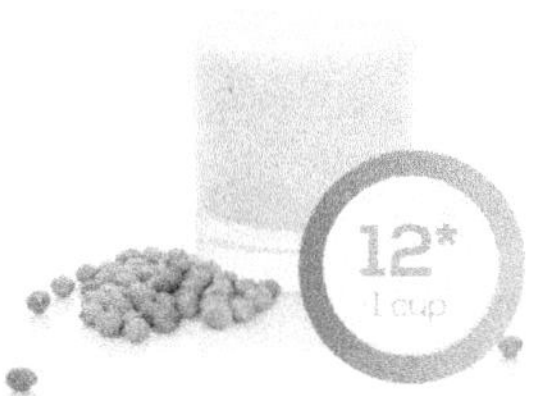

12*
1 cup

Soy milk

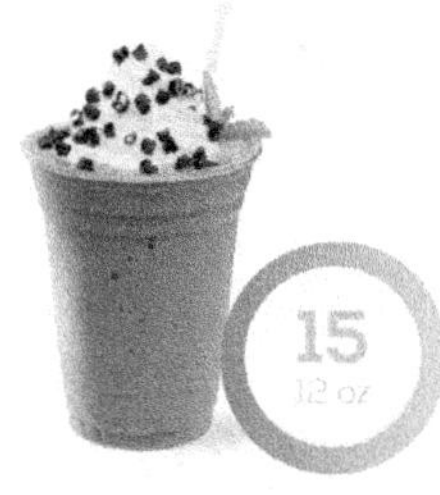

15
12 oz

Caffè latte

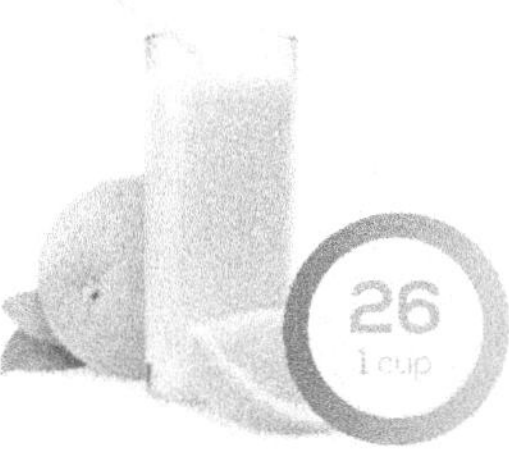

26
1 cup

Orange juice

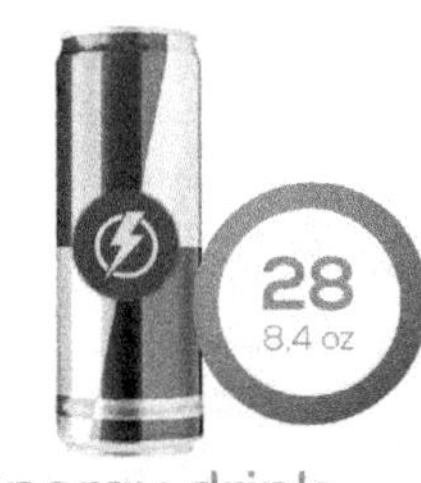

28
8.4 oz

Energy drink

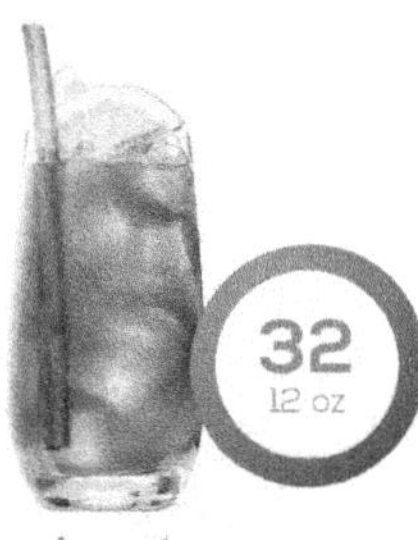

32
12 oz

Ice tea

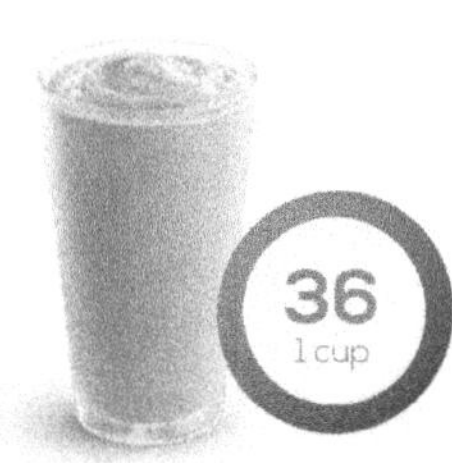

36
1 cup

Smoothie

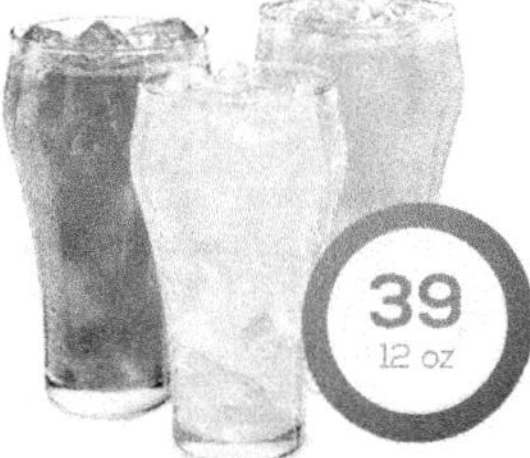

39
12 oz

Soft drink

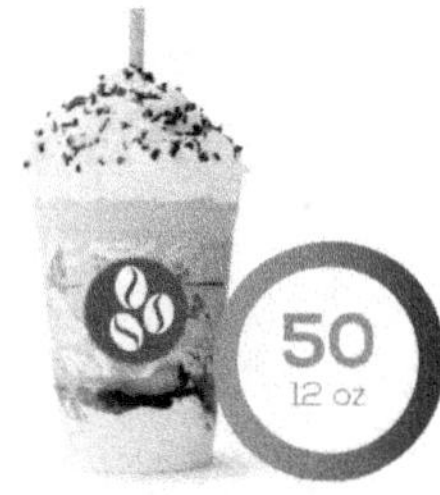

50
12 oz

Frappuccino

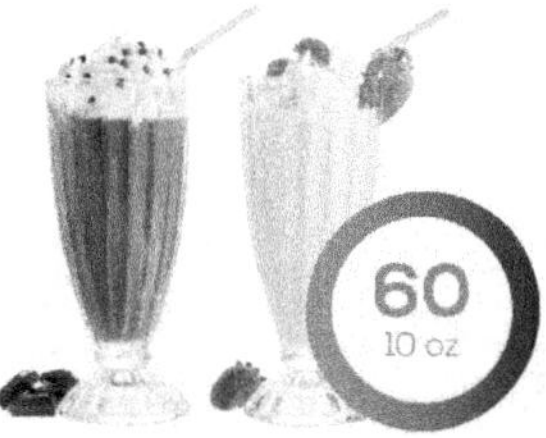

60
10 oz

Milkshake

BEST	← CARBS →	WORST

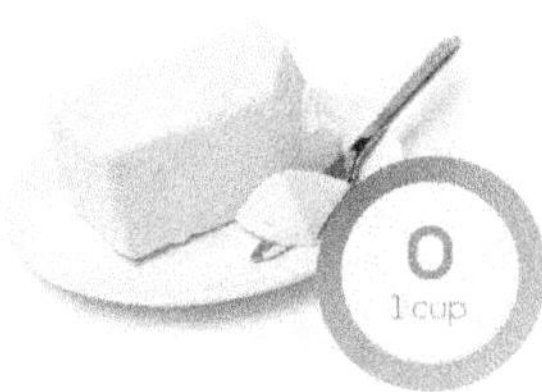

Butter

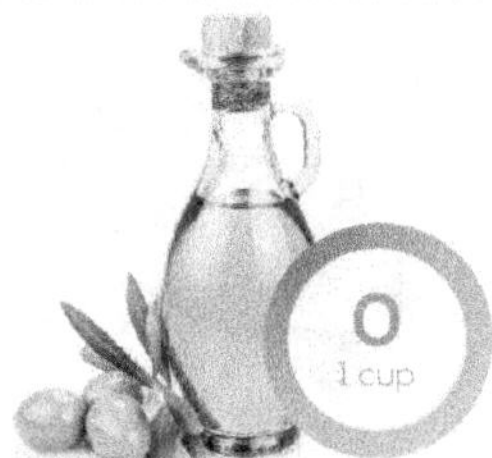

Olive oil

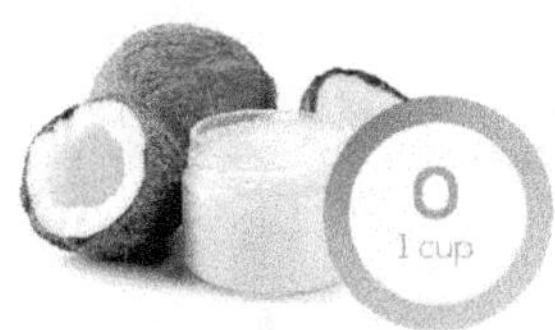

Coconut oil

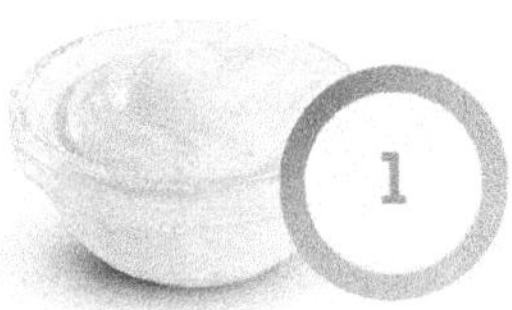

Mayonnaise

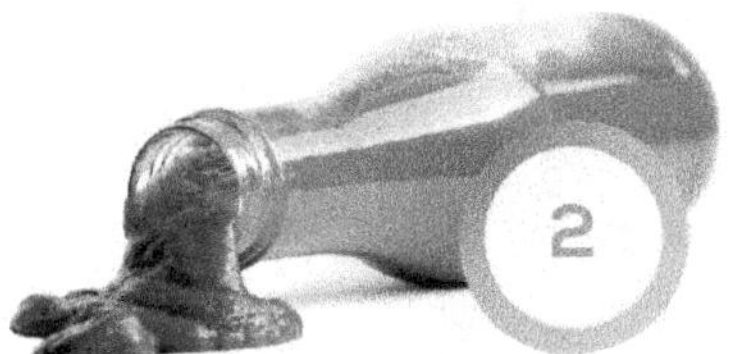

Tabasco / Hot sause

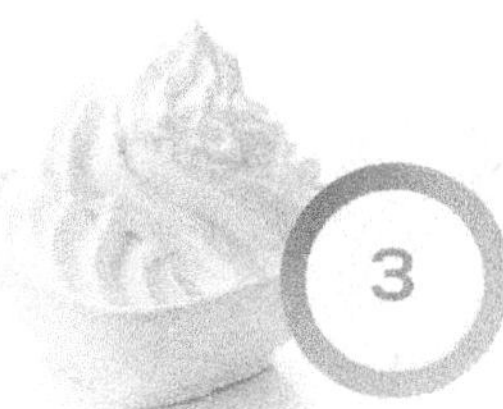

Heavy cream

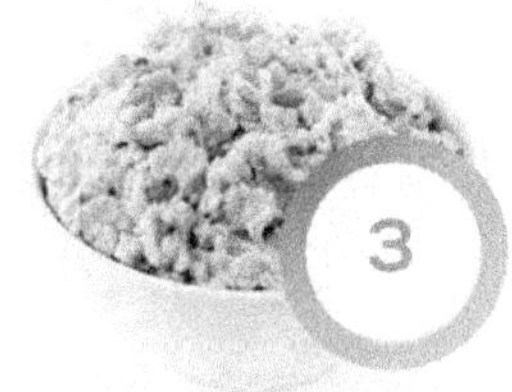

Guacamole

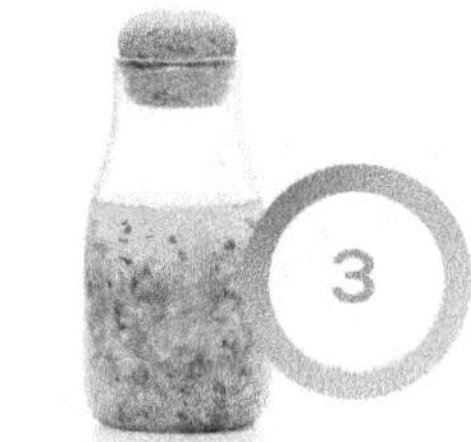

Vinaigrette

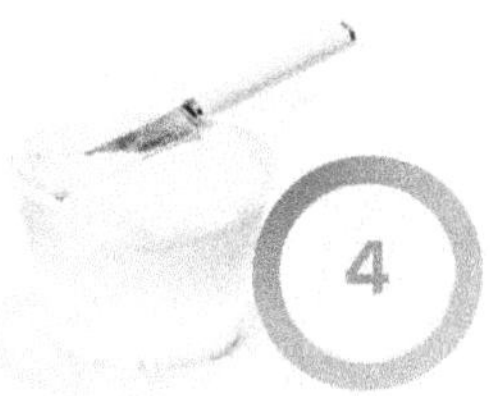

Cream cheese

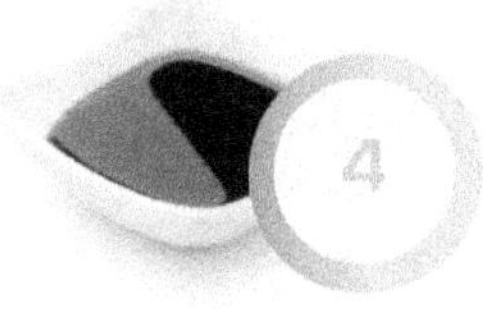

Soy sause

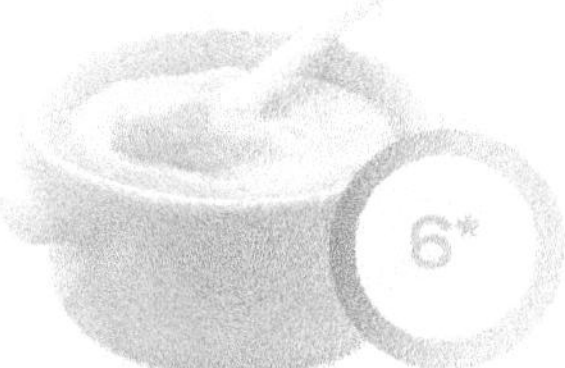

Mustard

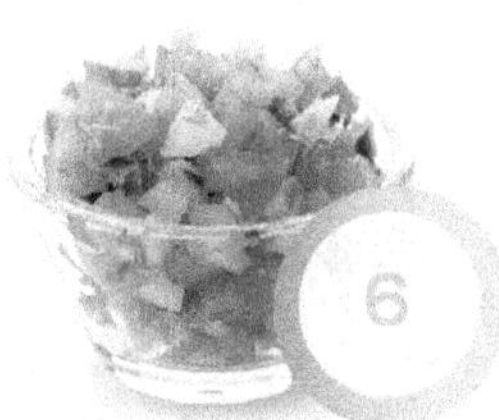

Salsa

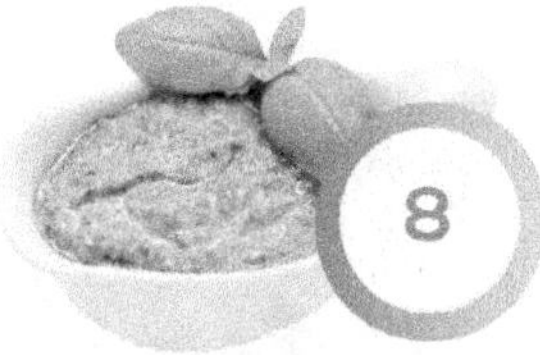

Pesto

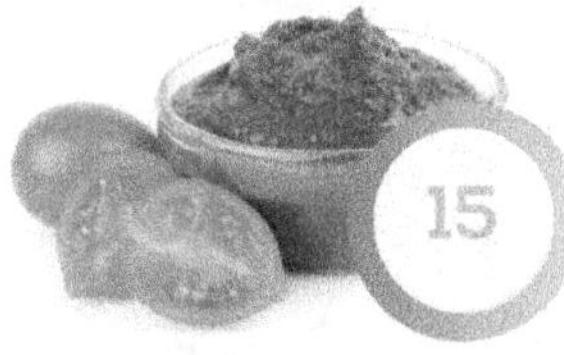

Tomato paste

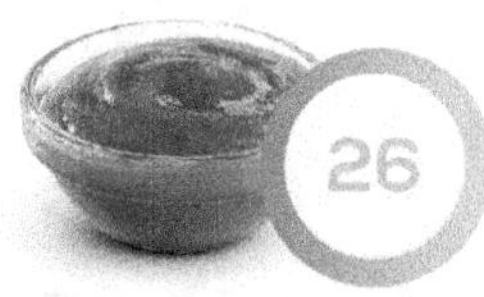

Ketchup

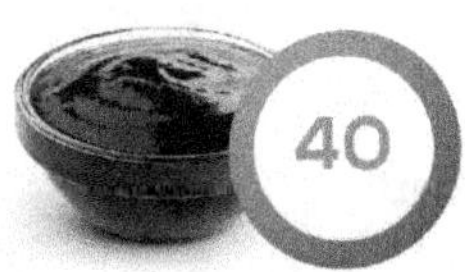

BBQ sause

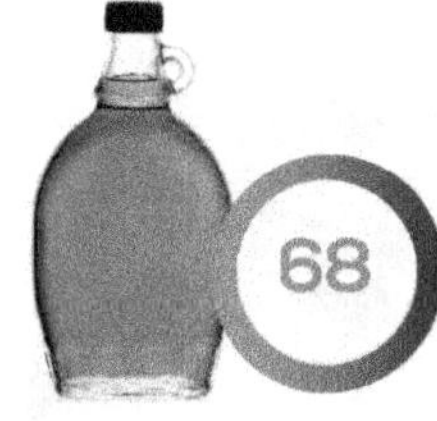

Maple syrup

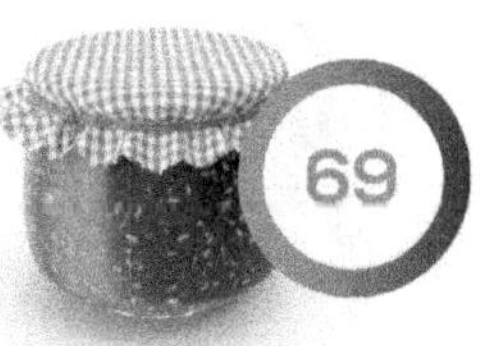

Jam

BEST	← CARBS →	WORST

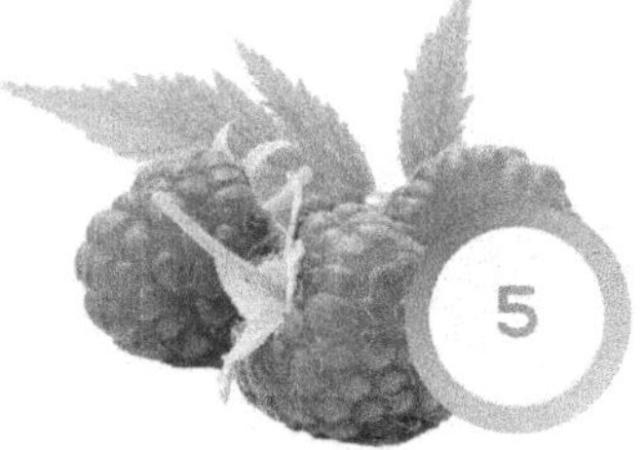

Raspberry

Blackberry

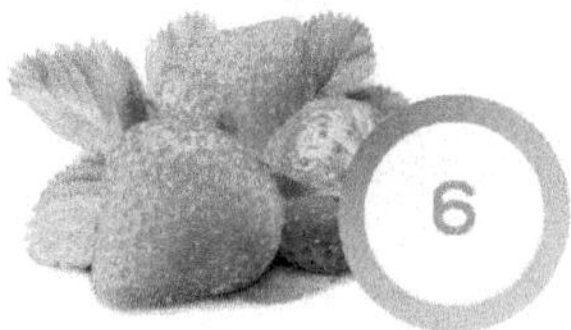

Strawberry

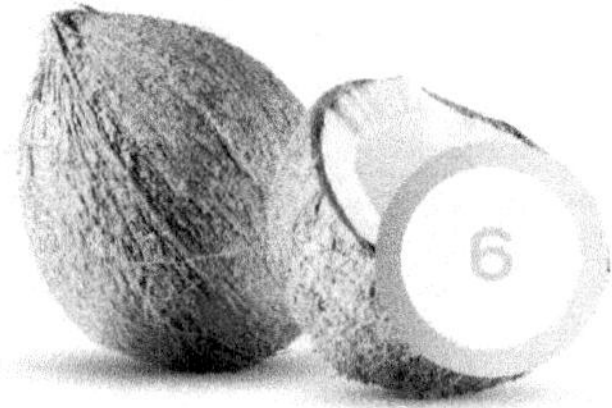

Coconut (Meat)

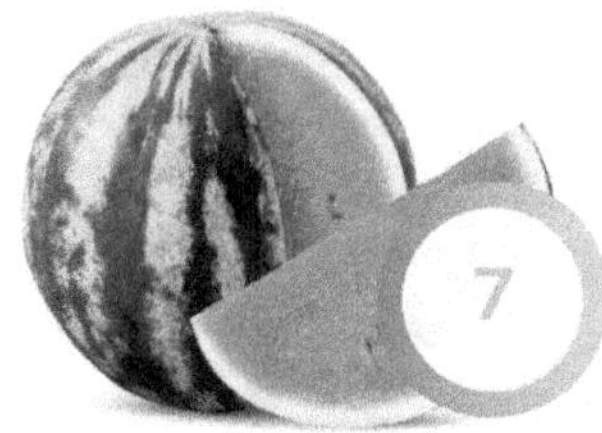

Watermelon

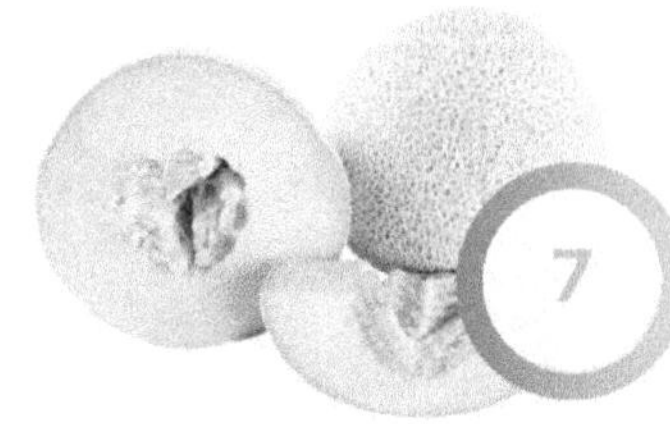

Cantaloupe

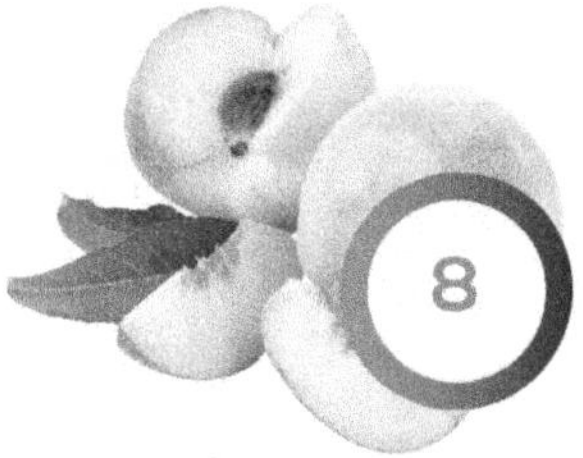

Peach

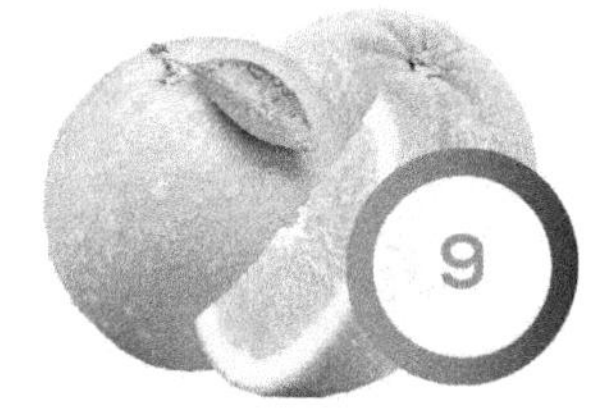

Orange

Plum

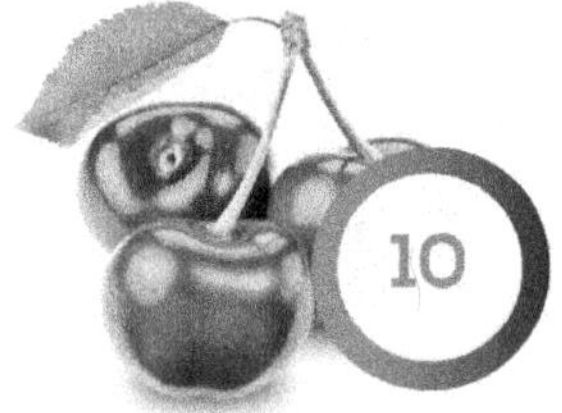

Cherries

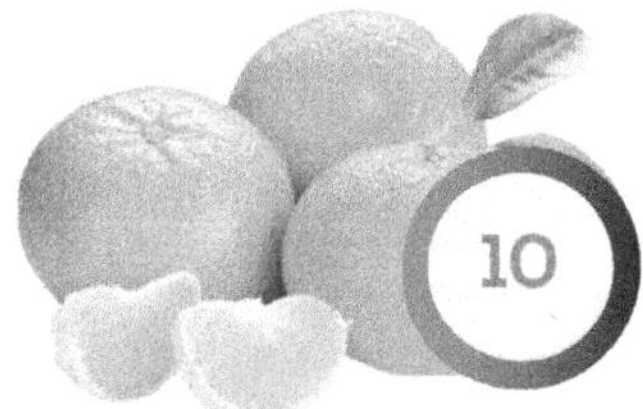

Clementine

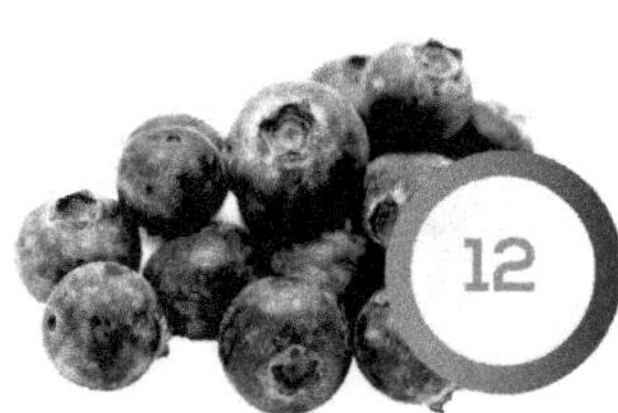

Blueberry

Pear

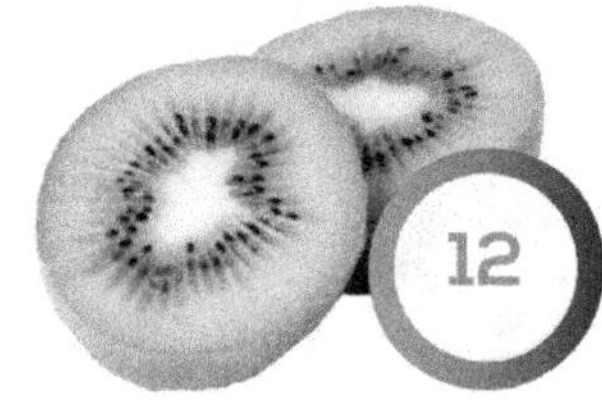

Kiwi

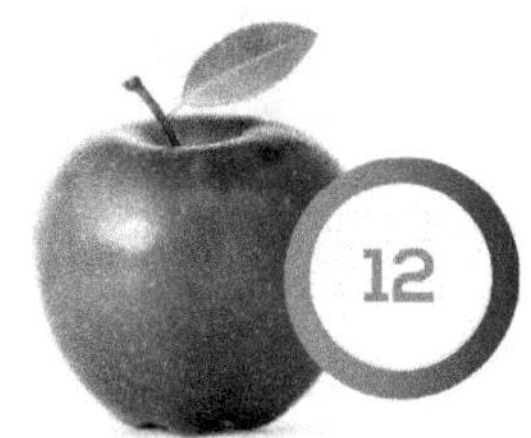

Apple

Pineapple

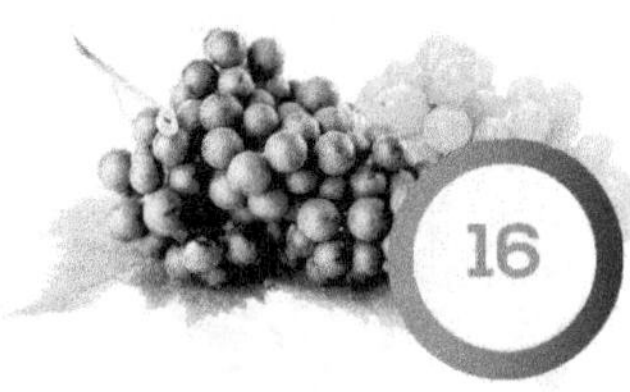

Grapes

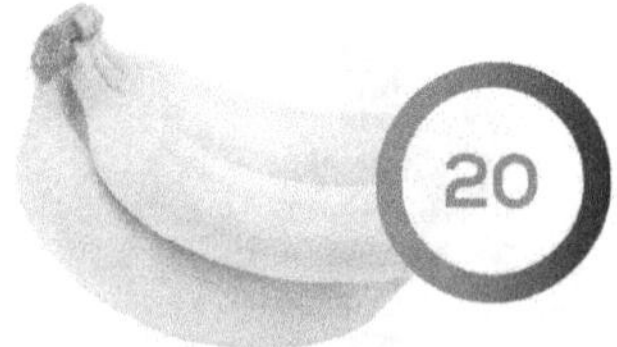

Banana

BEST ← **CARBS** → **WORST**

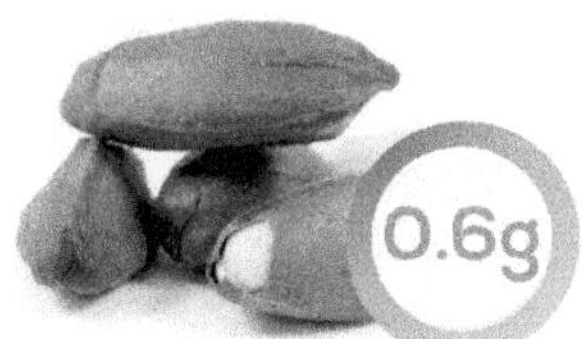

0.6g

Pili nuts

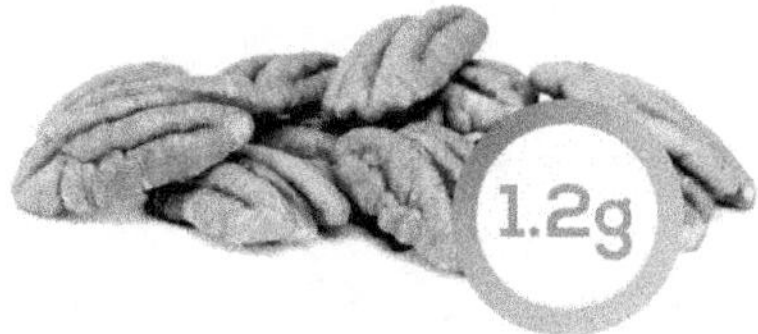

1.2g

Pecan

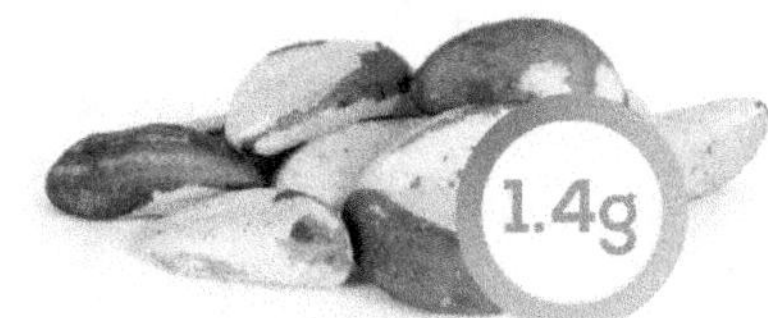

1.4g

Brazil nuts

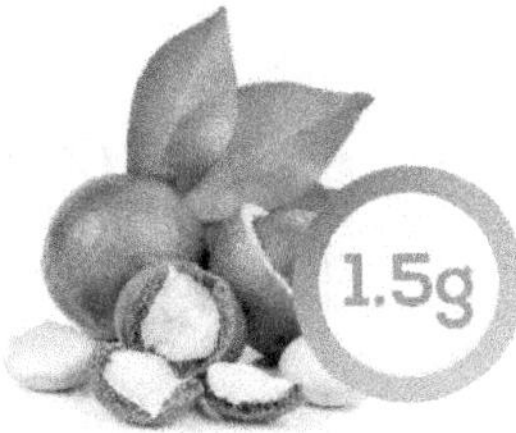

1.5g

Macadamia

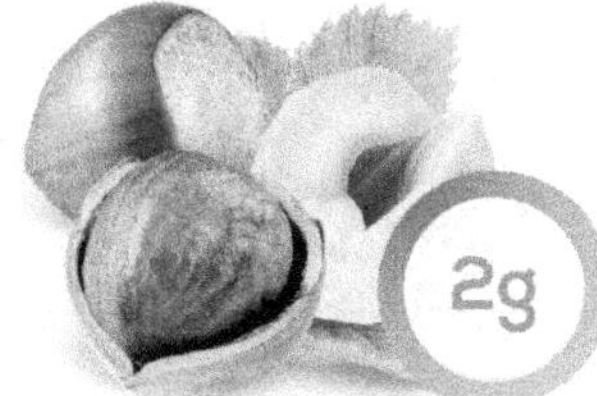

2g

Hazelnut

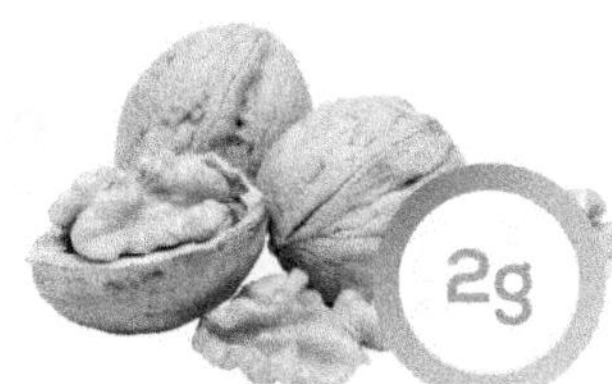

2g

Walnut

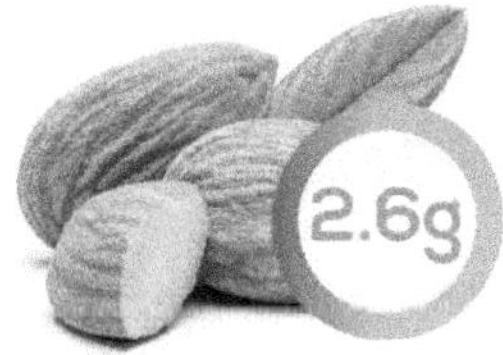

2.6g

Almonds

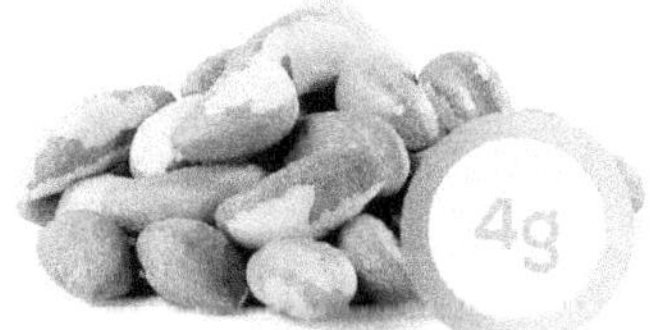

4g

Brazil

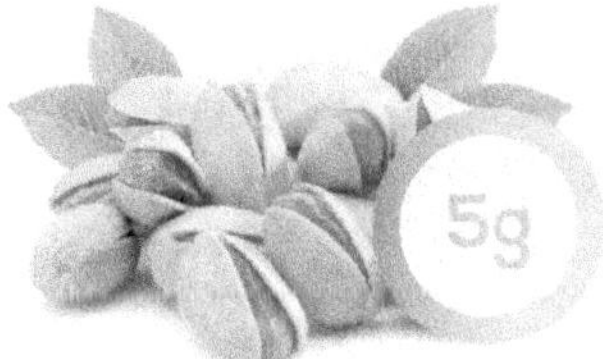

5g

Pistachio

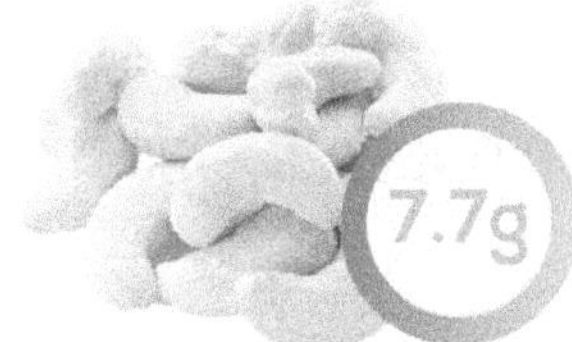

7.7g

Cashews

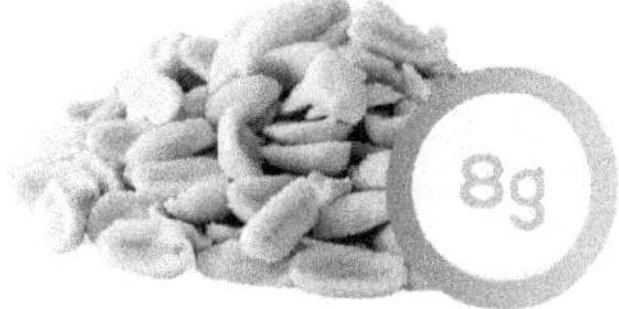

8g

Peanut

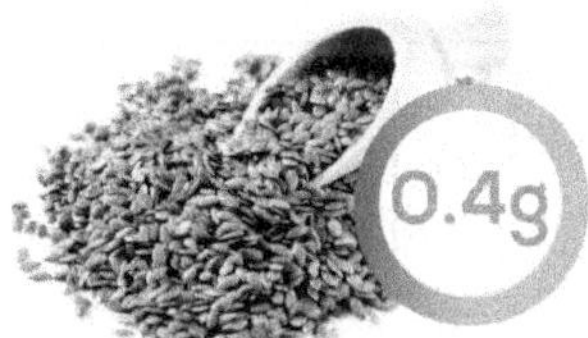

0.4g

Flax seeds

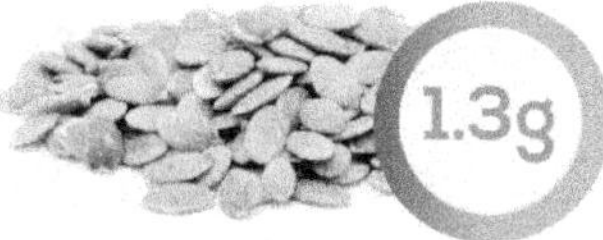

1.3g

Pumpkin seeds

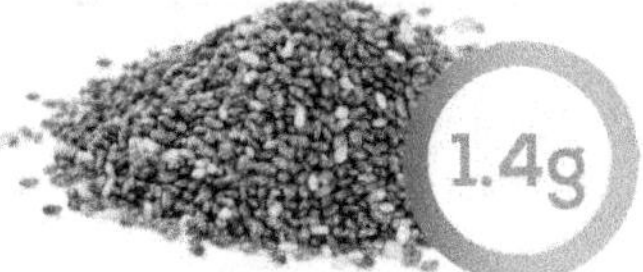

1.4g

Chia seeds

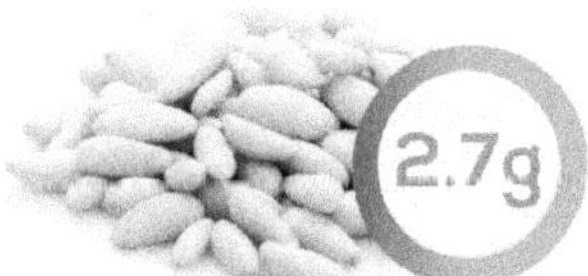

2.7g

Pine seeds

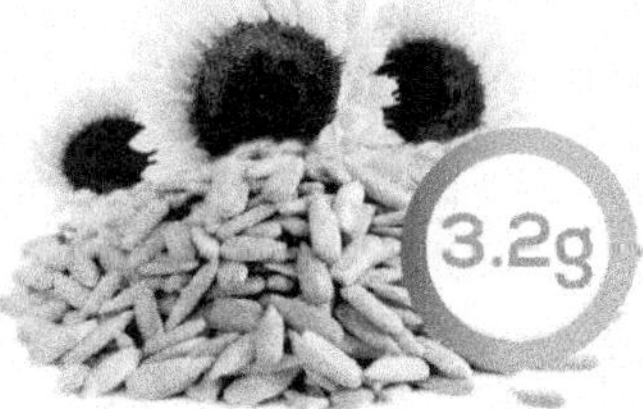

3.2g

Sunflower seeds

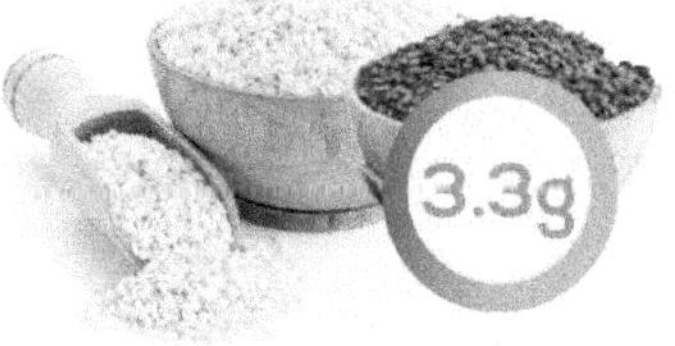

3.3g

Sesame seeds

LOW CARB SUGAR CONVERSION CHART

ERYTHRITOL	1 TBSP + 1 TSP	1/3 CUP	2/3 CUP	1 1/3 CUP
LIQUID STEVIA	1/16 TSP 6 DROPS	1/4 TSP 24 DROPS	1/2 TSP 48 DROPS	1 TSP 96 DROPS
STEVIA POWDER	1/16 TSP	1/4 TSP	1/2 TSP	1 TSP
TRUVIA ERYTHRITOL + STEVIA	1.5 TSP	1 TBSP + 2 TSP	3.5 TBSP	1/3 CUP + 1.5 TBSP
LIQUID MONK FRUIT	10 DROPS	40 DROPS	80 DROPS	160 DROPS
SWERVE ERYTHRITOL + OLIGOSACHARIDES	1 TBSP	1/4 CUP	1/2 CUP	1 CUP
ALLULOSE	1 TBSP + 1 TSP	5 TBSP + 1 TSP	1/2 CUP + 3 TBSP	1 1/3 CUP
XYLITOL	1 TBSP	1/4 CUP	1/2 CUP	1 CUP

Shopping List

BEEF	POULTRY	PORK	SEAFOOD	
• Steak	• Chicken	• Bacon	• Salmon	• Lobster
• Prime Rib	• Quail	• Ground pork	• Tuna	• Crab
• Veal	• Turkey	• Sausage	• Trout	• Bass
• Roast Beef	• Organs	• Bratwurst	• Cod	• Scallops
• Brisket	• Eggs	• Pork rinds	• Sardines	• Mussels
• Loin		• Ham	• Tilapia	• Clams
• Ground beef		• Pork chops	• Shrimp	• Oysters
• Stew meats				
• Organs				

OTHER • Deli meats • Jerky sticks • Biltong • Salami • Goat • Lamb

LEAFY GREENS

- Spinach
- Kale
- Swiss chard
- Lettuce
- Bok choy
- Watercress
- Endive
- Dandelion greens

CRUCIFEROUS VEGGIES

- Broccoli
- Cauliflower
- Red cabbage
- Green cabbage
- Napa cabbage
- Brussels sprouts

ALL OTHER VEGETABLES AND GREENS

- Avocado
- Asparagus
- Celery
- Spring onion
- Fennel
- Radish
- Kohlrabi
- Jalapeño peppers
- Zucchini
- Eggplant
- Green peppers
- Other bell peppers
- Cucumbers
- Tomatoes
- Spaghetti squash
- Sauerkraut
- White mushrooms
- Portobello mushrooms
- Beetroot
- Brown onion
- Red onion
- Carrots
- Bean sprouts
- Artichoke
- Ginger
- Garlic
- Olives
- Basil
- Sage
- Parsley
- Chives
- Dill

FRUITS AND BERRIES

- Raspberries
- Blackberries
- Strawberries
- Coconut
- Lemon
- Lime
- Starfruit

FATS AND OILS

- Coconut oil
- Olive oil
- Avocado oil
- MCT oil
- Grass fed butter

DAIRY

- Greek yogurt
- Kefir
- Heavy cream
- Half n' Half
- Feta
- Mozzarella
- Cheddar
- Blue cheese
- Parmesan
- Cottage cheese
- Swiss cheese
- Gouda
- Cream cheese
- Colby
- Ricotta
- Brie
- Goat cheese
- Sour cream

DRINKS

- Spring water
- Sparkling water
- Tea
- Coffee
- Bone broth
- Greens
- MCT powder mix
- Coconut milk
- Almond milk

CONDIMENTS AND SAUCES

- Apple cider vinegar
- Balsamic vinegar
- Mustard
- Ketchup (sugar free)
- Avocado Mayonnaise
- Salsa
- Lemon juice
- Horseradish
- Lime juice
- Hot sauces
- Soy sauce
- Tabasco

HERBS AND SPICES

- Apple cider vinegar
- Himalayan pink salt
- Sea salt
- Black pepper
- Cilantro
- Cinnamon
- Turmeric
- Cayenne
- Cumin
- Basil
- Thyme
- Sage
- Oregano
- Dill
- Rosemary
- Chili powder
- Paprika

SWEETNERS

- Monk Fruit
- Xylitol
- Lakanto
- Swerve
- Erythritol
- Stevia
- Pyure
- Truvia

CHOCOLATE

- Cocoa Powder
- Cacoa Powder
- Sugar Free Cooking Chocolate
- Dark Chocolate

FLOURS

- Almond Meal
- Almond Flour
- Coconut flour
- Ground Hazelnut flour
- Ground Macadamia flour
- Ground Peanut flour
- Ground Chai Seeds
- Flaxseed Meal
- Sunflower seed meal

THICKENING AGENTS

- Oat Fiber
- Psyllium Husks
- Gelatin
- Glucomannan
- Collagen Protein Powder
- Inulin
- Xanthan gum

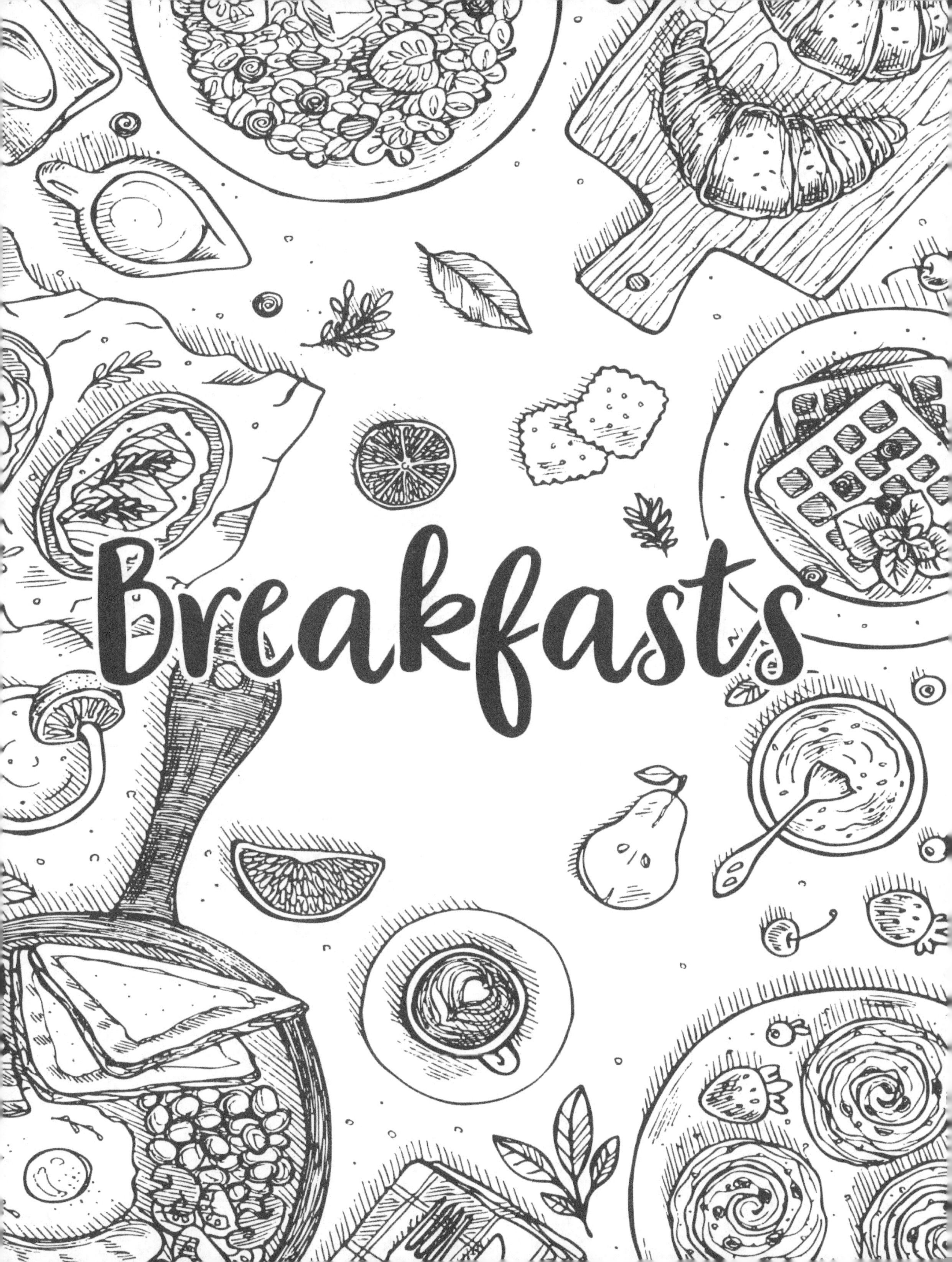
Breakfasts

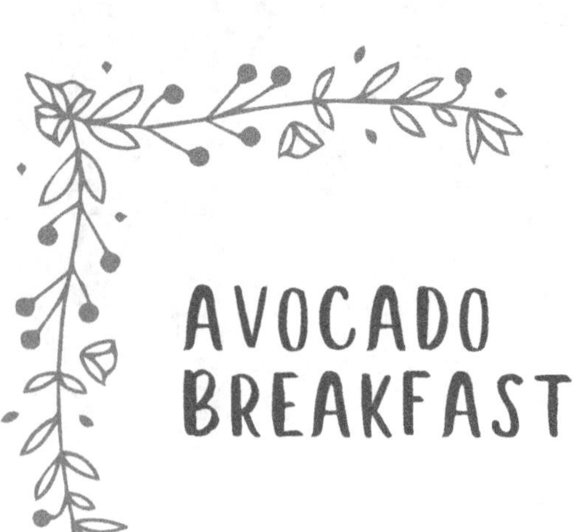

AVOCADO BREAKFAST CUPS

Ingredients

2 avocados, halved

2 tbsp salted butter

6 eggs

6 slices of bacon, chopped

Pinch of tomato paste or parsley for decoration

This is how you make the recipe

1. Scoop out most of the avocado flesh, leaving just a half-inch shell of avocado meat.
2. Warm up the butter in a saucepan.
3. In a bowl, mix the eggs with a pinch of salt and pepper.
4. Place the chopped pieces of bacon on one side of the pan and let them fry for a few minutes.
5. Add the eggs to the other side of the pan and scramble them.
6. Once both the bacon and eggs are done cooking, combine them and spoon into the avocado cups.
7. Decorate with parsley or tomato paste.

PORRIDGE

Ingredients

2 cups almond milk

1 cup almond flour

2 tbsp flax meal

2 tbsp chia seeds

2 tbsp coconut flakes

2 tbsp coconut oil

This is how you make the recipe

1. Combine all the ingredients in a pot. Stir while heating.
2. Bring to a simmer until it thickens up.
3. Pour into mugs and enjoy.

BLUEBERRY PANCAKES

Yield: 8	
Nutritional Values Per Serving:	
Net Carbs: 2 g	Protein: 12 g
Fat: 18 g	Calories: 258 kcal

Ingredients

3 eggs

1 cup almond milk

4 tbsp sweetener

2⅔ cups almond flour

½ cup blueberries

This is how you make the recipe

1. In a large bowl, whisk the eggs, almond milk and sweetener together until smooth.

2. Add the almond flour and whisk until you have a pancake batter.

3. Stir in the blueberries until well incorporated.

4. Heat up an oiled frying pan and when hot, portion out the pancakes and cook on both sides until golden.

BACON & EGG CASSEROLE

Servings: 8	
Nutritional Values Per Serving:	
Net Carbs: 2 g	Protein: 43 g
Fat: 38 g	Calories: 437 kcal

Ingredients

6 slices of bacon

12 eggs

½ cup soured cream

½ cup double cream

1¼ cups cheddar cheese, shredded

This is how you make the recipe

1. Preheat the oven to 350°F.

2. Cook bacon. After cooling down crumble into bits.

3. In a bowl, mix the eggs, sour cream, heavy cream, salt and pepper until well-combined.

4. Spread a layer of shredded cheddar to an oiled pan.

5. Pour the egg mixture on top of the cheese, then sprinkle crumbled bacon on top.

6. Bake for 30 minutes.

7. After removing it from the oven, you can garnish the casserole with green onions or herbs.

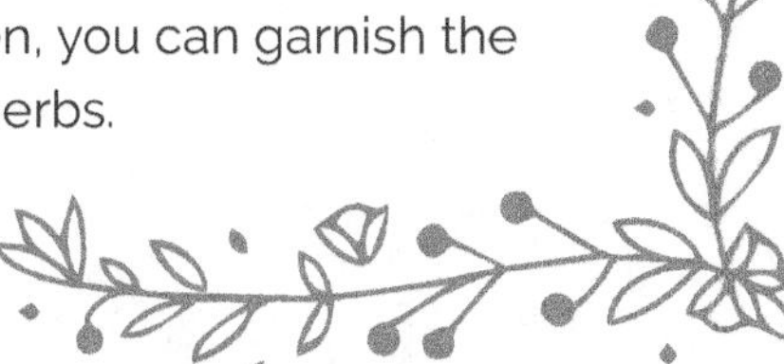

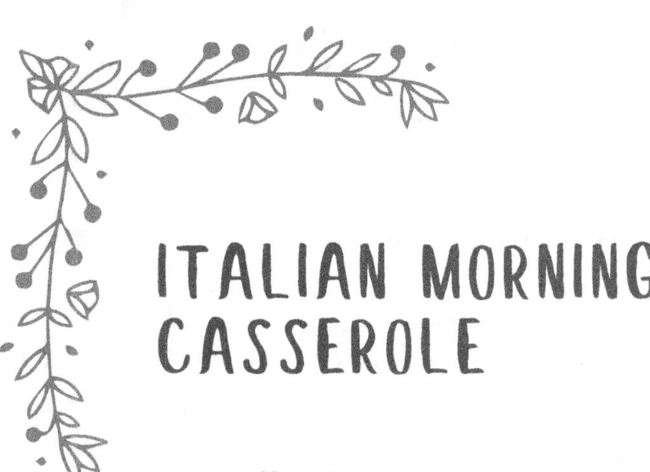

ITALIAN MORNING CASSEROLE

Ingredients

2 cups sausage, chopped

1½ cups Roma tomatoes, chopped

2 cups mozzarella, shredded

6 eggs

½ cup heavy cream

This is how you make the recipe

1. Preheat the oven to 350°F.

2. Fry the chopped sausage until done, then move it into a baking dish.

3. Add the tomatoes and cheese.

4. Mix the eggs with the double cream and pour over the casserole mixture.

5. Bake the casserole for 30-40 minutes.

EGG POCKETS

Ingredients

¾ cup mozzarella, shredded

⅓ cup almond flour

2 eggs

2 tbsp unsalted butter

3 slices of bacon

This is how you make the recipe

1. Preheat the oven to 400°F.

2. Melt the mozzarella and add the almond flour. Stir until well-combined.

3. Roll the dough out between 2 sheets of greaseproof paper.

4. Scramble the eggs and lay them with bacon slices in the middle of the dough.

5. Fold over and seal the edges of the dough.

6. With a fork, poke a few holes to release the steam

7. Bake for 20 minutes or until they turn golden brown.

8. Remove from the oven and enjoy!

CHOCOLATE COCONUT SMOOTHIE

Servings: 2

Nutritional Values Per Serving:
Net Carbs: 8 g   Protein: 26 g
Fat: 38 g   Calories: 500 kcal

Ingredients

1½ cups coconut milk

4 tbsp cocoa powder

2 tsp sweetener

Handful of ice cubes

4 scoops collagen protein

This is how you make the recipe

1. In a food processor, mix all the ingredients, except for the collagen, until well-combined.

2. Add the collagen and continue mixing slowly until all is combined.

3. Pour into two tall, chilled glasses and enjoy.

SPINACH BACON & EGG SALAD

Servings: 4   Serving size: 2½ cups

Nutritional Values Per Serving:
Net Carbs: 4.3 g   Protein: 12 g
Fat: 20 g   Calories: 248 kcal

Ingredients

1 clove garlic

12 cups spinach, chopped

4 eggs, hard-boiled and chopped

4 slices of bacon, cooked and crumbled

This is how you make the recipe

1. To make the dressing, mince the garlic and then smash it into a paste. Put in a small bowl.

2. Make a quick dressing with oil, vinegar, salt and pepper.

3. Place the spinach, eggs and bacon in a large bowl, then pour the dressing over the salad. Toss to combine.

4. For taste, you can sprinkle on any variety of available herbs such as thyme, oregano, basil, chives, etc.

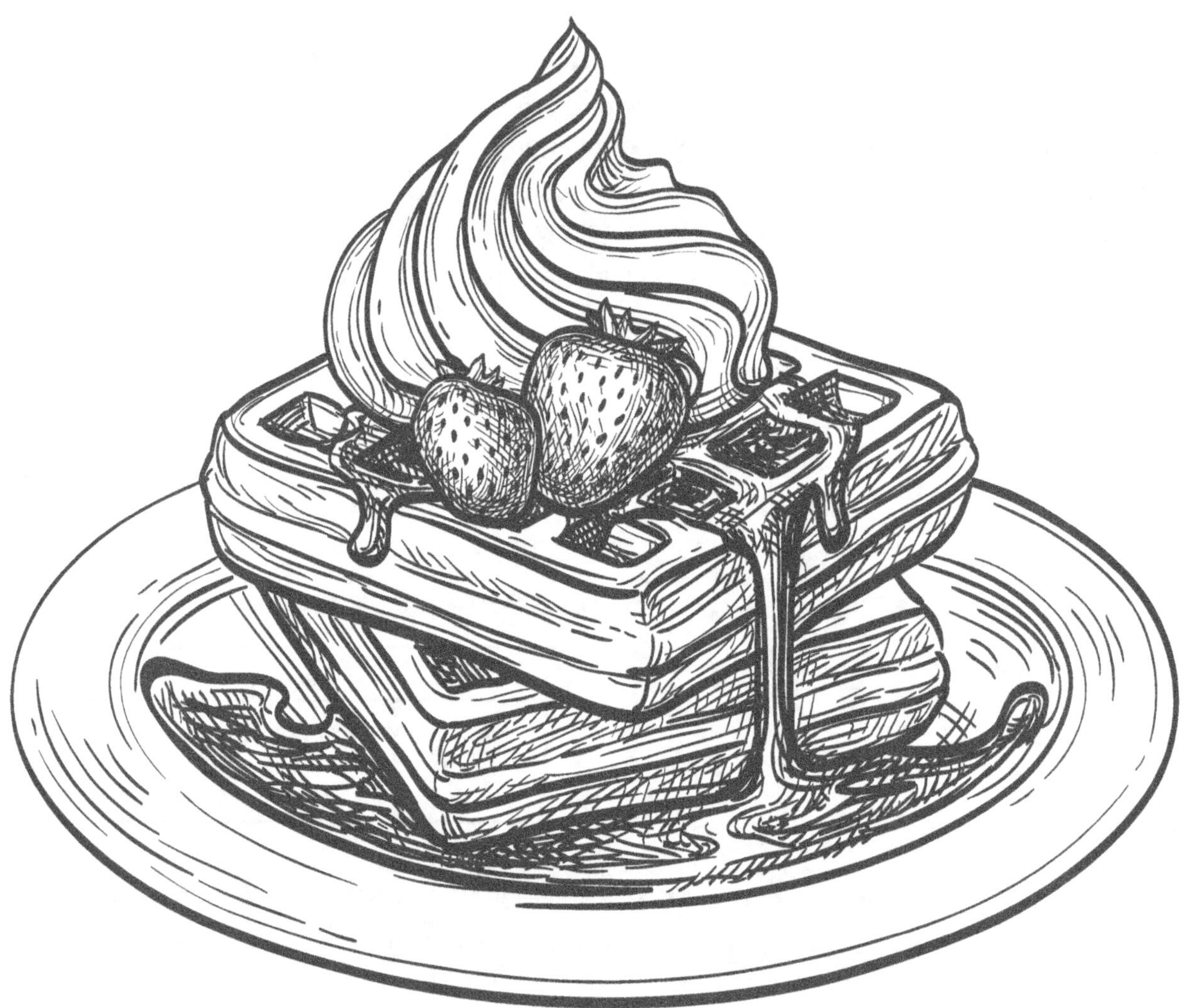

CHOCOLATE CHIP WAFFLES

Servings: 4

Nutritional Values Per Serving:

Net Carbs:	4.5 g	Protein:	34 g
Fat:	26 g	Calories:	400 kcal

Ingredients

4 scoops vanilla protein powder

4 large eggs

4 tbsp butter

¼ cup baking chocolate, grated

4 tbsp confectioners' sweetener

This is how you make the recipe

1. Separate the eggs.

2. Whisk the egg whites until stiff peaks form.

3. Combine the protein powder, egg yolks and the butter in a mixing bowl and whisk.

4. Fold the egg whites into this mixture, then add the chocolate and a pinch of salt.

5. Cook the batter in the waffle maker.

6. Sprinkle with confectioners' sweetener. Enjoy!

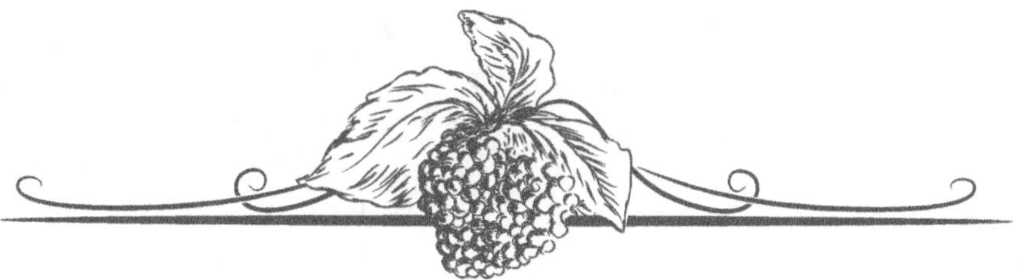

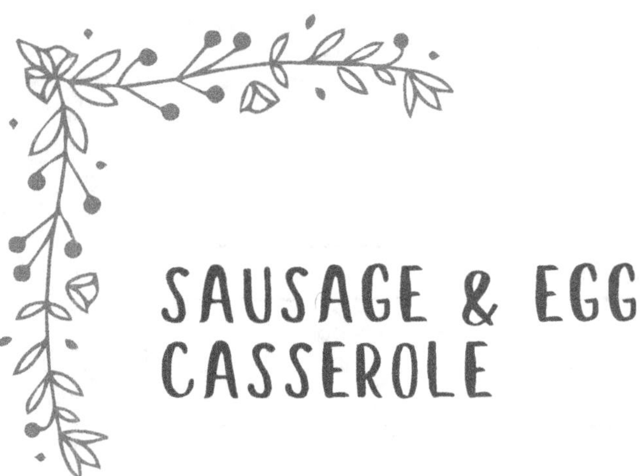

SAUSAGE & EGG CASSEROLE

Ingredients

16 slices breakfast sausage

10 eggs

½ cup heavy cream

1½ cups Cheddar cheese, shredded

2 tbsp parsley, chopped

This is how you make the recipe

1. Preheat the oven to 350˚F.

2. Heat an oiled pan over medium heat.

3. Add the sausage and cook, stirring until the sausage is browned and crumbled.

4. In a bowl, whisk the eggs, heavy cream, parsley and 1 cup of the Cheddar. Add salt and pepper to taste.

5. Lay out the sausage in an oiled baking dish.

6. Pour the egg mixture over the sausage slices.

7. Sprinkle with the remaining Cheddar.

8. Bake for 40 minutes.

9. Sprinkle with parsley and serve.

HAM & CHEESE PASTRY

Ingredients

¾ cup mozzarella, shredded

1 tbsp cream cheese

4 tbsp flax meal

2 slices of ham

2 slices of Provolone cheese

This is how you make the recipe

1. Preheat the oven to 400˚F.

2. Melt the mozzarella and cream cheese in a double boiler.

3. Add the flax meal and stir until well-combined.

4. Roll the dough out between 2 sheets of parchment paper.

5. Add the slices of ham and cheese.

6. Fold them over and seal the edges.

7. With a fork, poke a few holes to release the steam.

8. Bake for 20 minutes or until golden brown.

9. Remove from the oven and let cool.

BREAKFAST HASH BROWNS

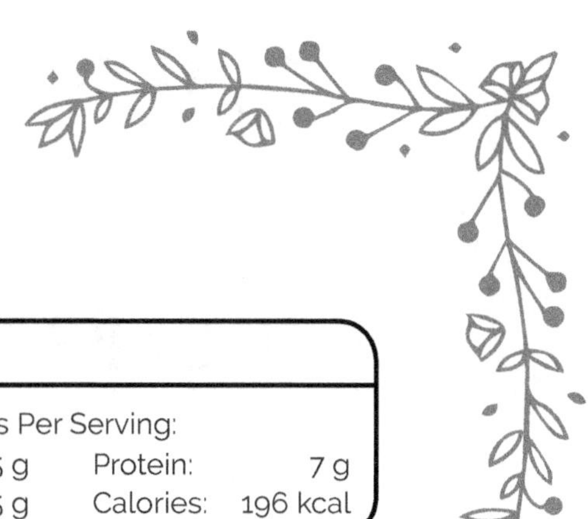

Servings: 4

Nutritional Values Per Serving:

Net Carbs:	5 g	Protein:	7 g
Fat:	15 g	Calories:	196 kcal

Ingredients

20 radishes, shredded

3 cups cauliflower, riced

3 cloves garlic, minced

½ tsp smoked paprika

6 strips bacon

This is how you make the recipe

1. In a large mixing bowl, combine the radishes, cauliflower and paprika. Salt and pepper to taste.

2. Mix until well-combined.

3. Fry the bacon until crispy, then crumble it into bits.

4. Heat an oiled pan over medium-high heat. Spread the hash mixture out evenly.

5. Sprinkle the bacon bits over the hash.

6. Fry the hash for 30 minutes until it is crispy. Stir and flip as needed.

BREAKFAST BARS

Servings: 6

Nutritional Values Per Serving:

Net Carbs:	3 g	Protein:	5 g
Fat:	33 g	Calories:	327 kcal

Ingredients

⅓ cup macadamia nuts

½ cup almond butter

¼ cup coconut oil

6 tbsp shredded coconut

¼ cup sweetener

This is how you make the recipe

1. Crush the macadamia nuts into bits.

2. Combine the almond butter, coconut oil and coconut in a mixing bowl.

3. Add the macadamia nuts and sweetener.

4. Mix until well-combined and pour the batter into a baking dish lined with greaseproof paper.

5. Refrigerate overnight.

6. Slice and enjoy.

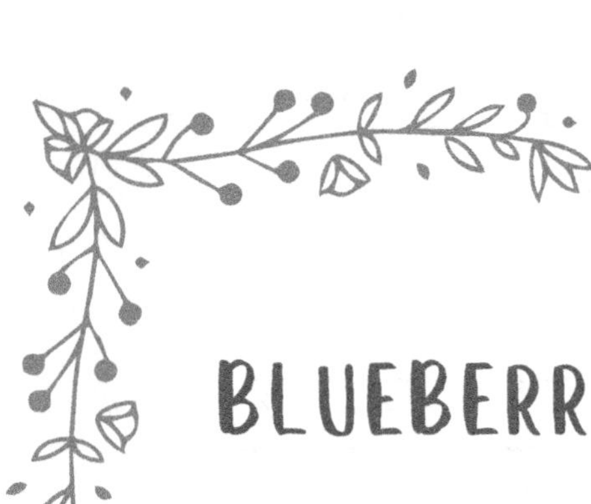

BLUEBERRY MUFFINS

Servings: 6

Nutritional Values Per Serving:
Net Carbs: 2.6 g   Protein: 5.6 g
Fat: 7.9 g   Calories: 105 kcal

Ingredients

3 eggs
¼ cup heavy cream
⅓ cup sweetener
5 tbsp coconut flour
½ cup fresh blueberries

This is how you make the recipe

1. Preheat the oven to 350°F. Line a muffin pan with cupcake papers.

2. In a bowl, whisk the eggs together with the cream and sweetener until well mixed.

3. Add the coconut flour to the egg mixture and whisk until smooth.

4. Let the batter thicken for 5 minutes. Then add the blueberries and mix well.

5. Fill six muffin cups.

6. Bake for 30 minutes.

7. Let cool and serve.

CREAM CHEESE WAFFLES

Servings: 12

Nutritional Values Per Serving:
Net Carbs: 1 g   Protein: 6 g
Fat: 19 g   Calories: 201 kcal

Ingredients

3 tsp cooking oil
12 eggs
¾ cup mayonnaise
3 tbsp almond flour
6 tbsp cream cheese

This is how you make the recipe

1. Coat the waffle iron with oil.

2. Blend the eggs, almond flour and mayonnaise until it becomes smooth.

3. Cut cream cheese into small ½-inch size cubes.

4. Pour the batter onto the hot waffle iron. Place a few cream cheese cubes evenly across the iron. Then close the iron.

5. Cook for 3-5 minutes, or until the waffle appears golden.

6. Remove the waffle from the iron.

7. Serve with confectioners' sweetener.

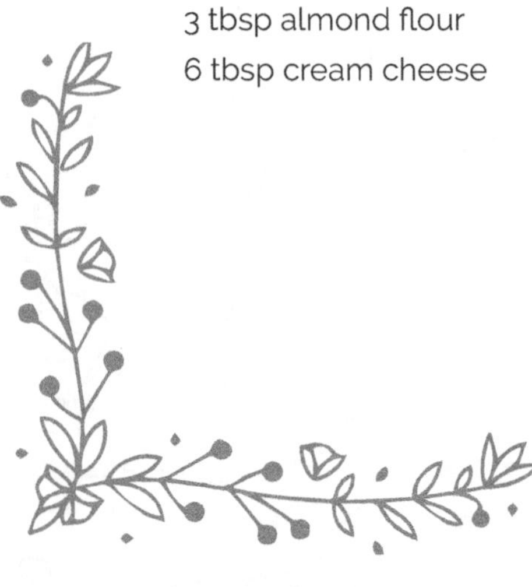

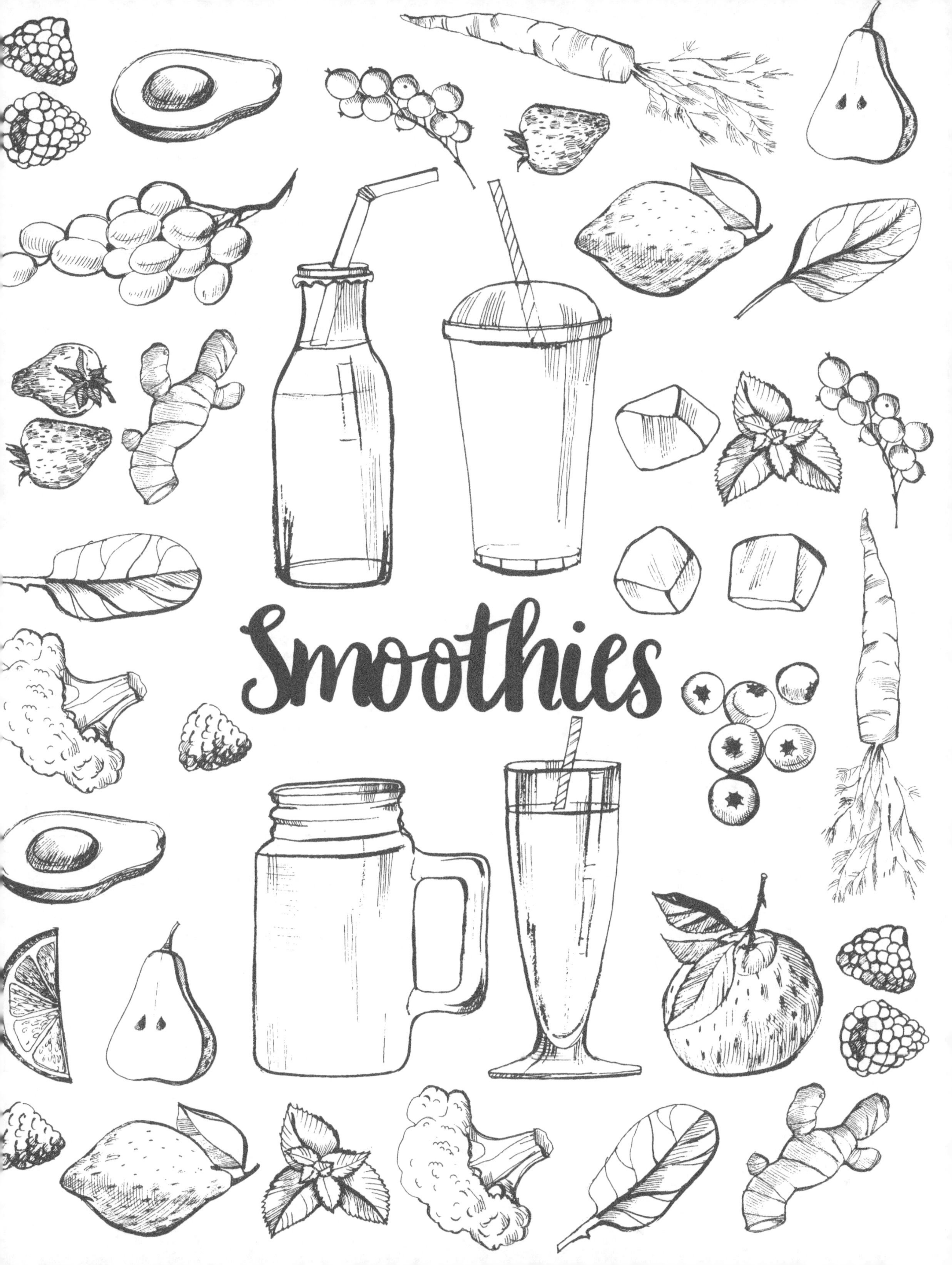
Smoothies

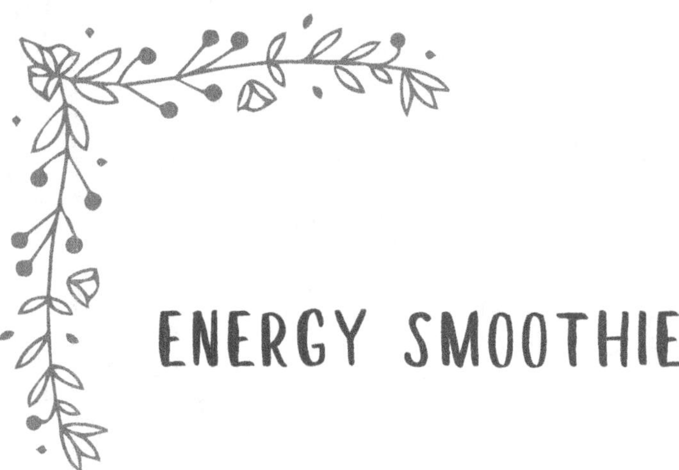

ENERGY SMOOTHIE

Ingredients

1 cup coconut milk

1 tsp cinnamon

2 tbsp ground chia seeds

½ cup whey protein

2 tbsp collagen powder

This is how you make the recipe

1. Add all of the ingredients in a blender along with a cup of cold water and 2 tbsp of coconut oil and mix until smooth.

2. Serve and enjoy!

PURPLE HEAVEN SHAKE

Ingredients

2 cups milk

6 tbsp unsweetened cocoa powder

1 cup berries (your choice)

1 tbsp chia seeds

2 tbsp confectioners' sweetener

This is how you make the recipe

1. Simply mix everything in a blender.

2. Serve and sprinkle with confectioners' sweetener.

MINTY GREEN SMOOTHIE

Servings: 2
Nutritional Values Per Serving:

Net Carbs:	4 g	Protein:	28 g
Fat:	15 g, 23%	Calories:	293 kcal

Ingredients

2 cups spinach

1 avocado

6 drops peppermint extract

3 tbsp whey protein powder

1 cup almond milk

This is how you make the recipe

1. Mix all the ingredients in a blender.

2. Drop in a cup of ice, sweeten to taste and blend.

3. Optional: You can add a tsp of lime juice and zest to perk it up even more!

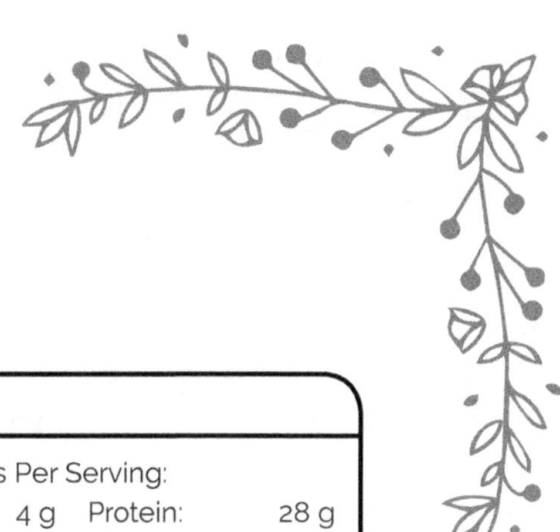

BLUEBERRY– VANILLA SHAKE

Servings: 2
Nutritional Values Per Serving:

Net Carbs:	3 g	Protein:	31 g
Fat:	21 g	Calories:	343 kcal

Ingredients

2 cups coconut milk

½ cup blueberries

2 tsp vanilla extract

2 tsp MCT oil

2 scoops protein powder

This is how you make the recipe

1. Put all the ingredients into a mixer, and blend until smooth.

2. Serve and enjoy!

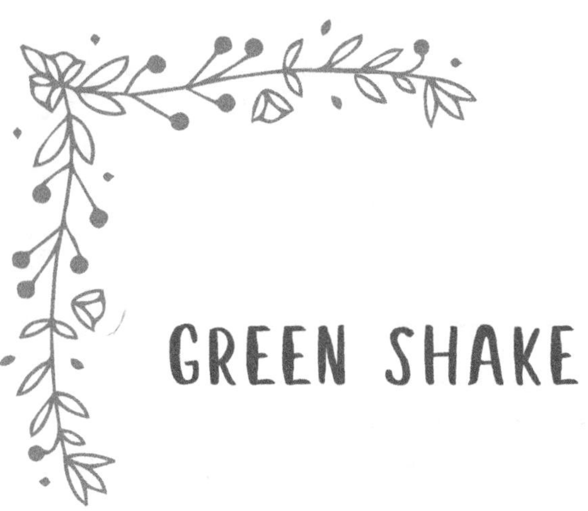

GREEN SHAKE

Servings: 2	Serving size: 1 tall glass
Nutritional Values Per Serving:	
Net Carbs: 3 g	Protein: 40 g
Fat: 27 g	Calories: 485 kcal

Ingredients

2 tbsp flax seed powder

2 tbsp chia seeds

1 scoop whey protein powder

2 cups frozen spinach

5 ice cubes

This is how you make the recipe

1. Combine all ingredients in a blender with 3 cups of water and mix for one minute.

2. Pour into glasses and enjoy!

ALMOND SMOOTHIE

Servings: 2	
Nutritional Values Per Serving:	
Net Carbs: 7.1 g	Protein: 10.7 g
Fat: 41.3 g	Calories: 453 kcal

Ingredients

2 cups almond milk

1 avocado

6 tbsp sweetener

4 tbsp almond butter

2 tbsp unsweetened cocoa powder

This is how you make the recipe

1. Place all ingredients into a blender with a cup of crushed ice and blend until smooth.

2. Pour into glasses and enjoy!

MINT SMOOTHIE

Servings: 1

Nutritional Values Per Serving:
Net Carbs: 4 g Protein: 1 g
Fat: 23 g Calories: 223 kcal

Ingredients

¾ cup coconut milk

½ cup almond milk

5 mint leaves

1 tbsp lime juice

This is how you make the recipe

1. Mix all of the ingredients until completely pureed.

2. Serve and enjoy.

PEANUT BUTTER CHOCOLATE MILKSHAKE

Servings: 4

Nutritional Values Per Serving:
Net Carbs: 3.1 g Protein: 3.6 g
Fat: 5.7 g Calories: 79 kcal

Ingredients

4 cups coconut milk

¼ cup sweetener

4 tbsp cocoa powder

4 tbsp peanut butter

Pinch of salt

This is how you make the recipe

1. Place all ingredients in a blender.

2. Blend until well-combined and frothy.

3. Serve and enjoy!

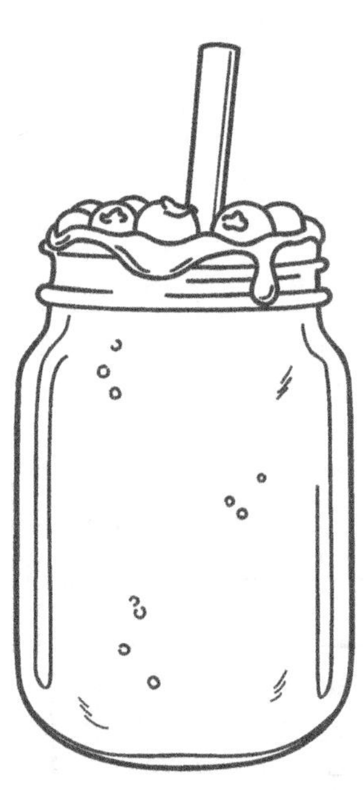

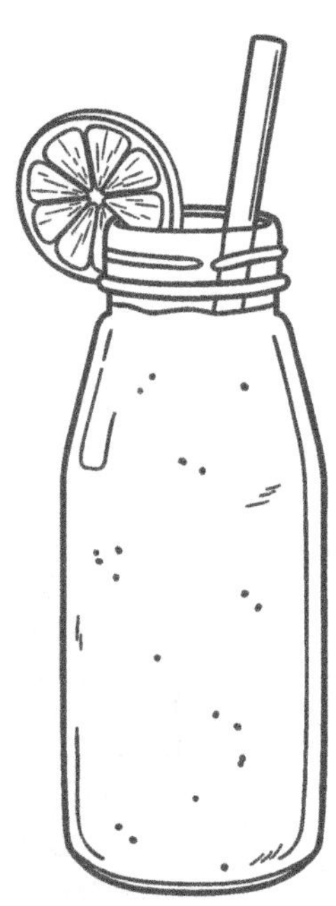

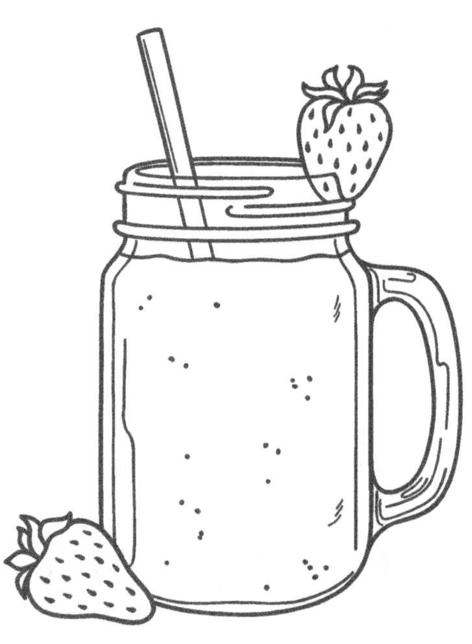

BLUEBERRY SMOOTHIE

Servings: 2

Nutritional Values Per Serving:
Net Carbs: 4 g Protein: 23 g
Fat: 10 g Calories: 215 kcal

Ingredients

2 cups coconut milk

½ cup blueberries

2 tsp vanilla extract

2 tsp coconut oil

¼ cup protein powder

This is how you make the recipe

1. Mix all the ingredients until smooth.
2. Serve and enjoy!

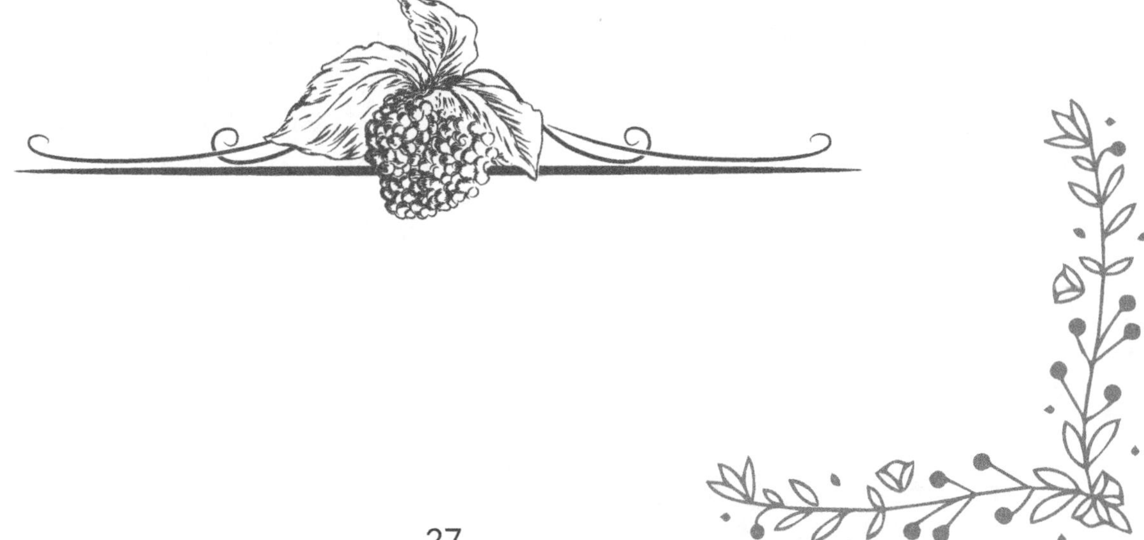

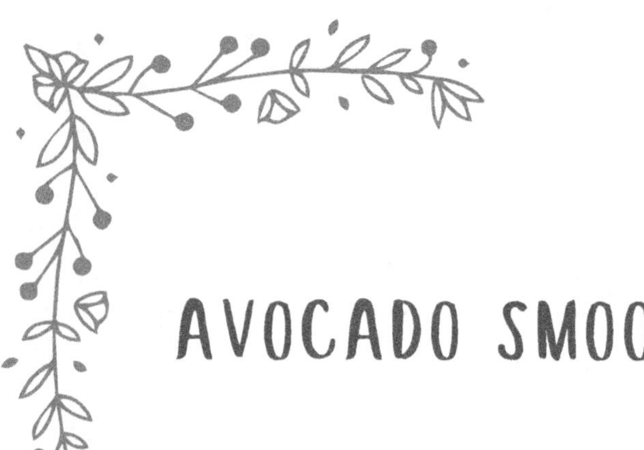

AVOCADO SMOOTHIE

Servings: 2

Nutritional Values Per Serving:
Net Carbs: 0.5 g   Protein: 1.4 g
Fat: 6.3 g   Calories: 240 kcal

Ingredients

½ avocado

1½ cups cold milk

1 tsp vanilla extract

2 tbsp sweetener

1 scoop protein powder

This is how you make the recipe

1. Blend all ingredients in a blender until completely smooth. Add a pinch of salt to taste.

2. Pour into glasses and enjoy!

COCOPUMPKIN SMOOTHIE

Servings: 2

Nutritional Values Per Serving:
Net Carbs: 2 g   Protein: 3 g
Fat: 24 g   Calories: 292 kcal

Ingredients

1 cup coconut milk

¼ cup pumpkin puree

2 tsp pumpkin pie spice

1 cup ice

This is how you make the recipe

1. Add coconut milk, pumpkin, pumpkin pie spice and ice to a blender.

2. Blend on high speed until smooth.

3. Pour into glasses and enjoy!

SHAMROCK SHAKE

Ingredients

1 cup coconut milk

½ avocado

1 tsp vanilla extract

1 large handful fresh mint leaves to taste

Sweetener to taste

This is how you make the recipe

1. Add all ingredients to the blender together with 1 cup of ice and blend until smooth.

2. Pour into glasses and enjoy!

BERRYCADO SMOOTHIE

Ingredients

⅔ cup strawberries, frozen

1 avocado

1½ cups coconut milk (use the one in carton)

1 tbsp lime juice

2 tsp sweetener

This is how you make the recipe

1. Add all ingredients with a half of a cup of ice into a blender.

2. Blend until smooth.

3. Pour into glasses and enjoy!

SUNFLOWER COCOA SHAKE

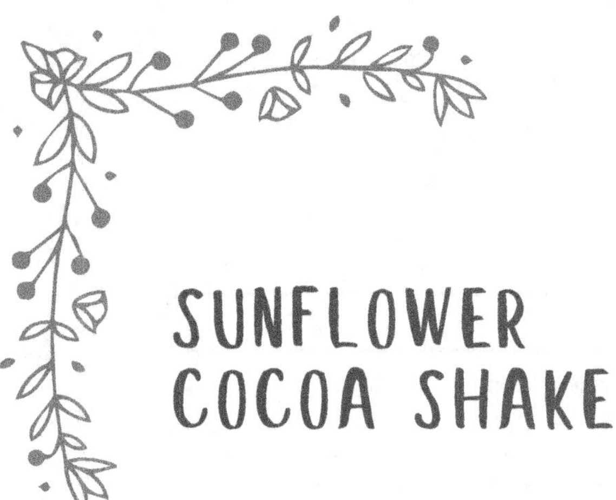

Yield: 2

Nutritional Values Per Serving:
Net Carbs: 3 g   Protein: 11 g
Fat: 24 g   Calories: 317 kcal

Ingredients

4 tbsp sunflower seed butter

⅔ cup coconut milk

1⅓ cup water

2 tsp cocoa powder

1 tsp vanilla extract

This is how you make the recipe

1. Combine all of the ingredients in a blender with 5 ice cubes.

2. Blend until smooth.

3. Serve and enjoy!

STRAWBERRY GREEN SMOOTHIE

Servings: 2

Nutritional Values Per Serving:
Net Carbs: 7 g   Protein: 1 g
Fat: 7 g   Calories: 106 kcal

Ingredients

36 strawberries, frozen

3 cups almond milk

2 avocados

½ cup confectioners' sweetener

2 whole strawberries, sliced, for decoration

This is how you make the recipe

1. Blend all ingredients until smooth.

2. Pour into two glasses.

3. Decorate with slices of strawberry.

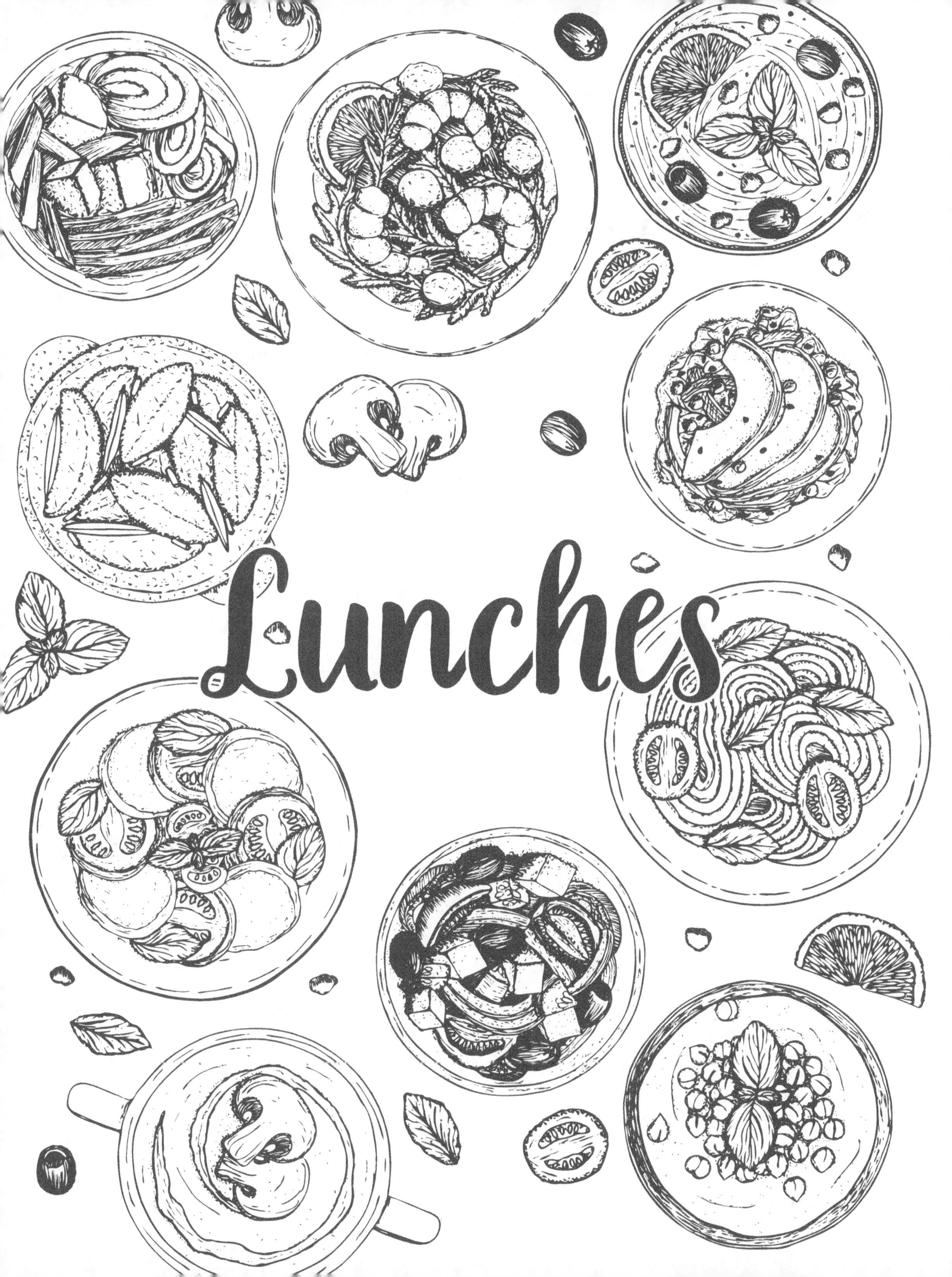
Lunches

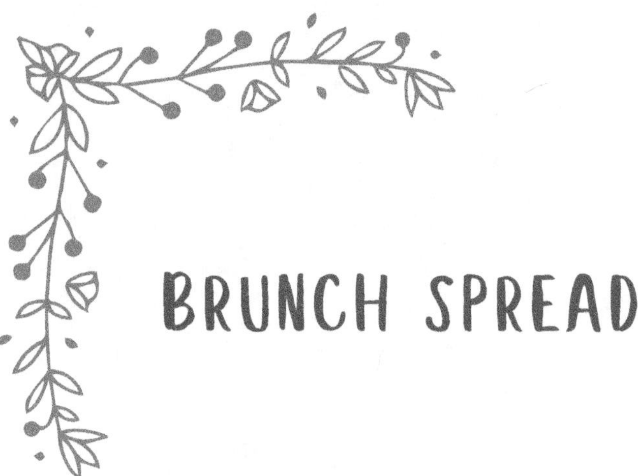

BRUNCH SPREAD

<table><tr><td colspan="2">Yield: 4</td></tr><tr><td colspan="2">Nutritional Values Per Serving:</td></tr><tr><td>Net Carbs: 6,14 g</td><td>Protein: 17 g</td></tr><tr><td>Fat: 38 g</td><td>Calories: 426 kcal</td></tr></table>

Ingredients

4 eggs

24 asparagus spears

12 slices of bacon

This is how you make the recipe

1. Preheat the oven to 400°F. .

2. Wrap two spears of asparagus together with a slice of bacon. Stretch it tight as you wind it.

3. Prepare a baking tray with parchment paper and lay out the asparagus rolls.

4. Bake for 20 minutes.

5. Soft boil the 4 eggs.

6. Cool off the soft-boiled eggs in ice water, then peel off the tops and place them in egg cups.

7. Scoop off the tops of the eggs, exposing the nice liquid yolks.

8. Dip the asparagus into the eggs and enjoy!

BACON CRANBERRY KALE

<table><tr><td colspan="2">Servings: 4</td></tr><tr><td colspan="2">Nutritional Values Per Serving:</td></tr><tr><td>Net Carbs: 8 g</td><td>Protein: 14 g</td></tr><tr><td>Fat: 73 g</td><td>Calories: 749 kcal</td></tr></table>

Ingredients

3½ cups kale

6 tbsp butter

12 slices of bacon

4 tbsp hazelnuts

½ cup cranberries

This is how you make the recipe

1. Chop the kale into large pieces.

2. Fry the bacon until crispy, then add the kale and cook for a few minutes. Salt and pepper to taste.

3. Sprinkle in the cranberries nut and stir. Enjoy!

MEXICAN CHEESE CRISPS

Servings: 2	Serving size: 12 crisps

Nutritional Values Per Serving:

Net Carbs:	0 g	Protein:	24 g
Fat:	36 g	Calories:	396 kcal

Ingredients

1 cup Cheddar cheese, shredded

2 medium sized jalapenos

4 slices of bacon

1 handful cilantro leaves

This is how you make the recipe

1. Preheat the oven to 425 ˚F and lay out parchment paper on a baking sheet.

2. Bake the bacon and crumble it.

3. Add a tbsp of shredded cheese on the greaseproof paper. Place a slice of jalapeno on top of it. Sprinkle with the crumbled bacon and a leaf of coriander .

4. Bake for 8 minutes.

5. Remove it and let cool down.

6. Enjoy!

CHICKEN SALAD

Servings: 4	

Nutritional Values Per Serving:

Net Carbs:	4 g	Protein:	28 g
Fat:	78 g	Calories:	837 kcal

Ingredients

4 boneless chicken thighs

6 slices of bacon

4 cherry tomatoes

½ head of romaine lettuce

¾ cup mayonnaise

This is how you make the recipe

1. Fry the bacon, then crumble it. Set aside

2. Fry the chicken until golden brown, shred it and add salt, pepper to taste.

3. Clean the lettuce, put it on plates and top with chicken, bacon, tomatoes, and mayonnaise.

4. Optional: You can add herbs and garlic.

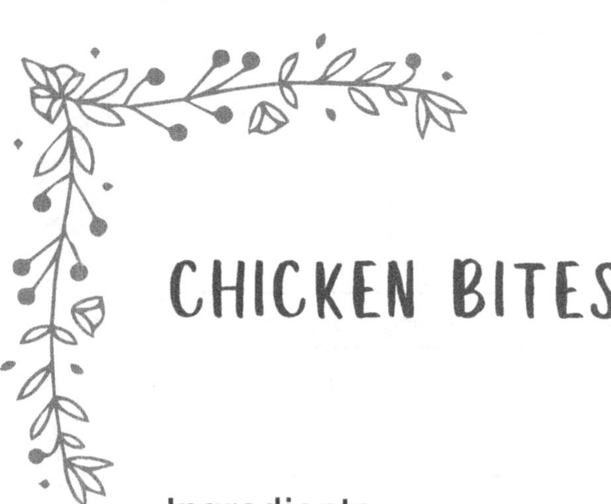

CHICKEN BITES

Yield: 18

Nutritional Values Per Piece:

Net Carbs:	3 g	Protein:	5 g
Fat:	2 g	Calories:	47 kcal

Ingredients

6 slices of bacon

2 boneless, skinless chicken breast halves, cubed

½ cup barbecue sauce

This is how you make the recipe

1. Preheat the oven to 400°F.

2. Cook the bacon until partially cooked, but not crisp.

3. Slice the bacon lengthwise to make 18 thin strips.

4. Place chicken cubes on a plate; sprinkle with salt, pepper and wrap a strip of bacon around each chicken cube; secure with a toothpick and lay it out on a parchment-lined baking sheet.

5. Bake for 18 minutes, until chicken is fully cooked.

6. If desired, add horseradish and sour cream to the sauce.

CUCUMBER BITES

Servings: 4   (20 nuggets 1 serving)

Nutritional Values Per Serving:

Net Carbs:	3 g	Protein:	7 g
Fat:	10 g	Calories:	140 kcal

Ingredients

1 large cucumber

1 small avocado

1 package smoked salmon

½ tsp sesame seeds

1 tsp herbs

This is how you make the recipe

1. Cut the smoked salmon pieces into 1-inch wide by 2-inch long pieces.

2. Slice the cucumbers into ¼-inch thick slices.

3. Cut the avocado into small pieces, similar in size to the cucumber slices.

4. Place one cucumber slice and one avocado onto a piece of salmon and wrap each of them up.

5. Sprinkle with sesame seeds and herbs. Enjoy!

CHEESEBURGER CASSEROLE

Servings: 6

Nutritional Values Per Serving:
Net Carbs: 4.9 g Protein: 30.5 g
Fat: 28.8 g Calories: 431 kcal

Ingredients

1 medium spaghetti squash

4 slices of bacon, chopped

1 lb. ground beef

1½ cups Cheddar cheese, shredded

2 cloves garlic, minced

This is how you make the recipe

1. Preheat the oven to 400°F and line a baking sheet with parchment paper. Cut the squash in half, scoop out the seeds and bake for 40 minutes.

2. Fry the bacon until crispy. Lay out on a paper towel.

3. Cook the minced beef until almost cooked through, add garlic. Add salt and pepper to taste.

4. Scoop the flesh out of the squash or courgette and mix it with the minced beef. Spread this mixture out over the bottom of a frying pan.

5. Sprinkle on the cheese, cover and reduce the heat to let it melt.

6. Sprinkle with the bacon and serve.

WRAPPED CHICKEN TENDERLOINS

Yield: 12 pieces

Nutritional Values Per Serving:
Net Carbs: 0.1 g Protein: 13 g
Fat: 15 g Calories: 204 kcal

Ingredients

Tenders:

12 chicken tenderloins

12 slices of bacon

Ranch Dip:

⅓ cup sour cream

⅓ cup mayo

4 tsp mixed herbs (i.e. garlic, onion, parsley, dill, etc.)

This is how you make the recipe

1. Preheat the oven to 400°F.

2. Wrap each chicken tender tightly with a slice of bacon.

3. Place them on a parchment-lined baking sheet. Bake for 35-45 minutes until the bacon is crispy and the chicken is fully cooked.

4. Meanwhile, combine the dip ingredients.

5. Dip the fillets and enjoy!

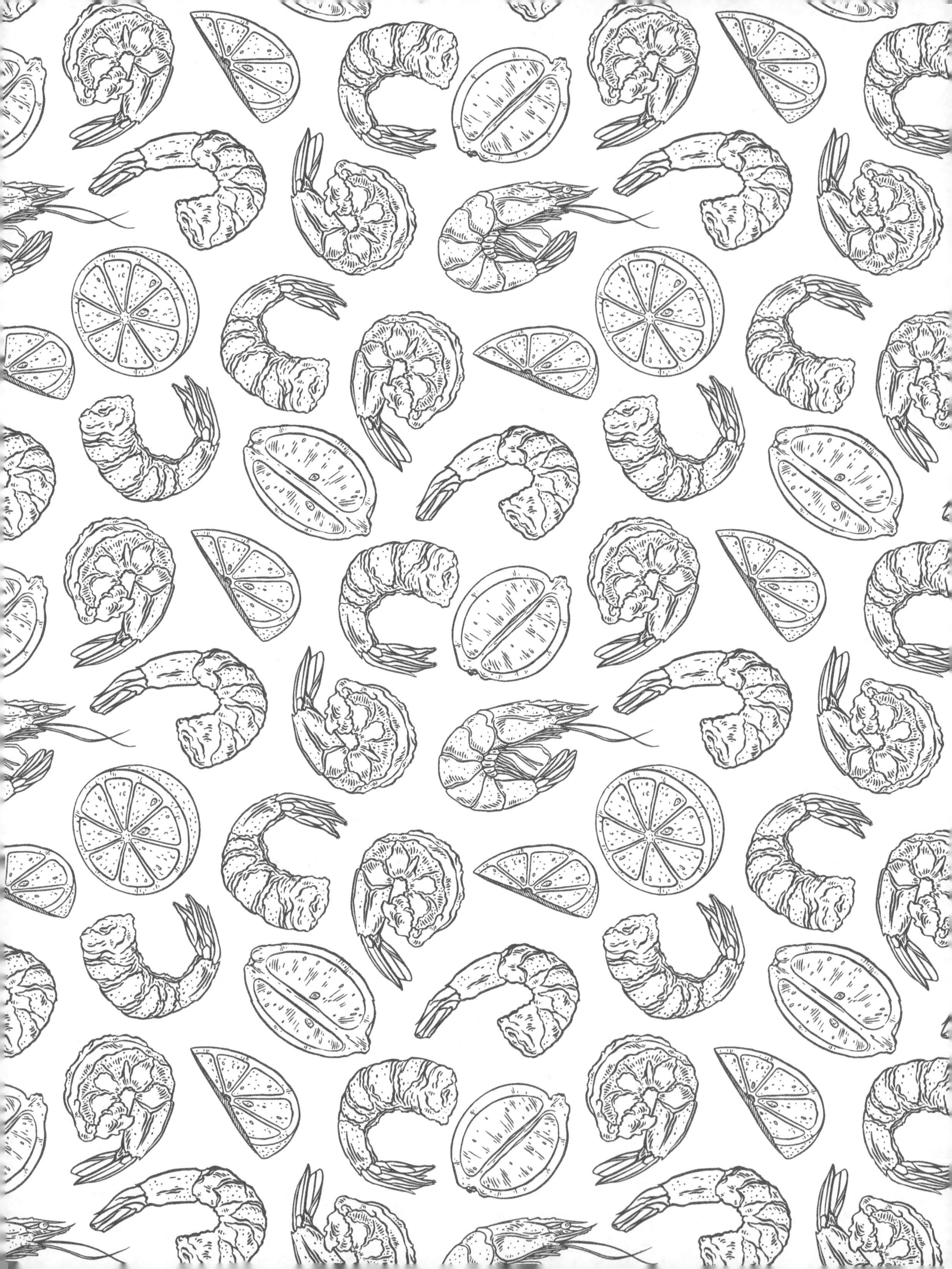

SHRIMP STACKS

Yield: 4

Nutritional Values Per Serving:
Net Carbs:	14.2 g	Protein:	12.3 g
Fat:	21.8 g	Calories:	289 kcal

Ingredients

12 shrimp, with tails

3 avocados

2 limes

4 leaves of basil

Coconut oil

This is how you make the recipe

1. Set the oven to broil. (500°F)

2. Line a baking sheet with parchment paper. Brush on coconut oil.

3. Arrange the shrimps on the sheet. Sprinkle with a little salt and drops of lime.

4. Broil the shrimp for 5 minutes.

5. Mix the avocado in a bowl with the rest of the lime juice and salt to taste.

6. After cooking, remove the shrimps from the oven.

7. Spoon the avocado mix on plates.

8. Add 3-4 shrimps on top of each avocado round and decorate with a basil leaf.

9. Serve and enjoy!

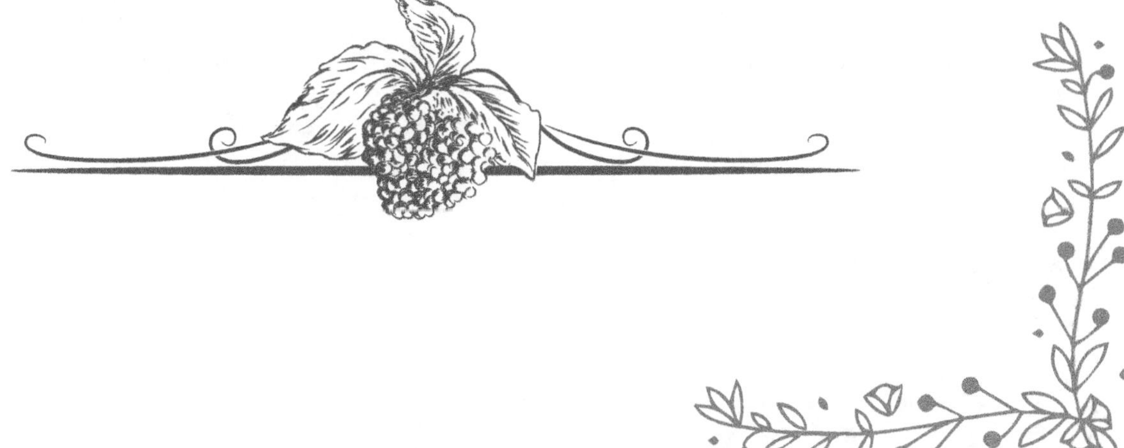

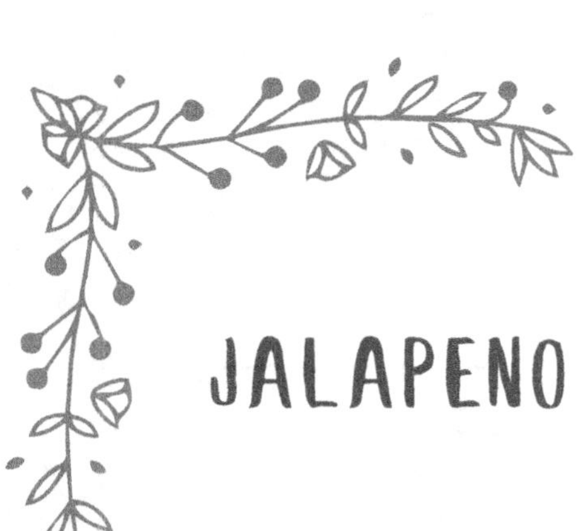

JALAPENO POPPERS

Yield: 16	Serving size: 1

Nutritional Values Per Serving:
Net Carbs: 1 g — Protein: 2.9 g
Fat: 6.6 g — Calories: 79 kcal

Ingredients

1 cup cream cheese

½ cup cheddar cheese, shredded

8 jalapenos, halved, de-seeded

8 slices of bacon, cut in half

1 tbsp rosemary

This is how you make the recipe

1. Preheat the oven to 375˚F and line a baking tray with parchment paper.

2. Fry the bacon slices for 3 minutes. Set aside.

3. In a double boiler, heat the cream cheese, the shredded cheddar, salt, and pepper.

4. Scoop the cream cheese mixture into the jalapeno's halves.

5. Wrap a slice of bacon around each jalapeno and pin it with a toothpick if needed.

6. Place jalapenos on the baking tray and bake for 15 minutes.

7. Then turn the oven to broil and cook for another 2-3 minutes.

NUT BUTTER BARS

Yield: 8 bars

Nutritional Values Per Serving:
Net Carbs: 2 g — Protein: 6 g
Fat: 28 g — Calories: 292 kcal

Ingredients

2 eggs

4 tbsp coconut oil

4 tbsp nut butter of your choice

1 cup macadamia nuts

¼ cup pumpkin seeds

This is how you make the recipe

1. Preheat the oven to 350˚F and line a baking dish with parchment paper.

2. Mix all ingredients until smooth. Pour into the dish.

3. Bake for 16-18 minutes.

4. Cool, refrigerate to harden, and cut into equal-size pieces. Enjoy!

WORCESTERSHIRE BURGERS

Servings: 4	
Nutritional Values Per Serving:	
Net Carbs: 2 g	Protein: 26 g
Fat: 40 g	Calories: 479 kcal

Ingredients

1 lb. ground beef

1 tbsp Worcestershire sauce

1 tbsp herbs

4 oz onion, sliced

1 clove garlic

This is how you make the recipe

1. Combine the minced beef with the Worcestershire sauce, herbs and garlic. You may wish to add a couple tablespoons of avocado or coconut oil.

2. Mix with your hands and form into four balls. Press these into burger patties.

3. Season the outside of the patties with a light sprinkling of salt and pepper and grill until done.

4. Heat the onions in a little oil in a pan. Add ½ teaspoon of sweetener and cook until beginning to caramelize. Enjoy!

PIZZA MUFFIN

Yield: 12	Serving: 6 (2 cups)
Nutritional Values Per Serving:	
Net Carbs: 4.4 g	Protein: 26.7 g
Fat: 30.4 g	Calories: 402.2 kcal

Ingredients

12 slices of ham

12 slices Italian sausage

12 tbsp pizza sauce

3 cups mozzarella cheese, grated

24 slices of pepperoni

This is how you make the recipe

1. Preheat the oven to 375˚F.

2. Brown the Italian sausage in frying pan.

3. Line a 12-cup muffin pan with ham slices. Divide sausage, pizza sauce, mozzarella cheese and pepperoni/salami slices between each cup.

4. To enhance the taste, you can sprinkle on minced garlic and herbs such as sage, basil and mint.

5. Bake for 10 minutes and grill for 1 minute.

6. Set the pizza muffin on a paper towel for a few minutes and enjoy!

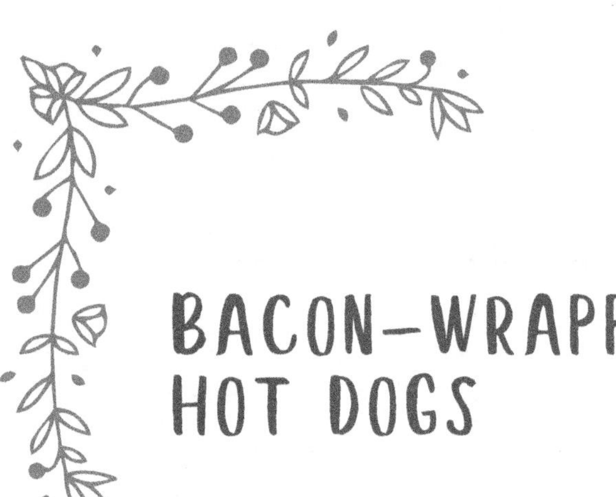

BACON-WRAPPED HOT DOGS

Yield: 8

Nutritional Values Per Serving:
Net Carbs: 2 g   Protein: 3 g
Fat: 4 g   Calories: 60 kcal

Ingredients

16 slices of bacon

8 beef hot dogs

⅓ cup mustard

¼ cup sweetener

1 clove garlic, minced

This is how you make the recipe

1. Preheat the oven to 400°F.

2. Cut bacon in half lengthwise and cook it until partially cooked but not crispy. Remove to paper towels to drain; keep warm.

3. Cut the hot dogs in quarters.

4. Wrap a thin slice of bacon around each piece of hot dog; secure with toothpicks. Place them in a baking dish.

5. Bake for 10 minutes and flip after 5 minutes.

6. In a bowl, combine the mustard, sweetener and garlic; drizzle over bacon-wrapped hot dogs.

7. Bake until bacon is crispy. Delicious!

HAM PICKLE WHEELS

Yield: 42

Nutritional Values Per Serving:
Net Carbs: 1 g   Protein: 2 g
Fat: 3 g   Calories: 34 kcal

Ingredients

1 cup cream cheese

10 slices Genoa salami

1 tbsp horseradish

7 slices of ham

14 pickles

This is how you make the recipe

1. In a food processor mix the cream cheese, salami and horseradish. You can even sprinkle on herbs if you wish.

2. Spread this onto the slices of ham.

3. Lay two pickles in the middle of each slice of ham. Roll the ham up tightly and refrigerate for a few hours.

4. Slice and serve.

CAESAR EGG SALAD LETTUCE WRAPS

Servings: 4

Nutritional Values Per Serving:

Net Carbs:	2.75 g	Protein:	13.5 g
Fat:	22 g	Calories:	254 kcal

Ingredients

6 eggs, hard-boiled

3 tbsp Caesar dressing

3 tbsp mayonnaise

½ cup Parmesan cheese, grated

4 large romaine lettuce leaves

This is how you make the recipe

1. In a bowl, combine chopped eggs, Caesar dressing, mayonnaise, half of the Parmesan cheese and pepper.

2. Place mixture onto romaine leaves and sprinkle with remaining Parmesan cheese. Add additional herbs to taste.

EGG-AVO SALAD WRAPS

Servings: 4

Nutritional Values Per Serving:

Net Carbs:	0 g	Protein:	5 g
Fat:	2 g	Calories:	136 kcal

Ingredients

4 eggs, hard-boiled

1 avocado

2 tsp lemon juice

3 tbsp mayonnaise

4 Boston lettuce leaves

This is how you make the recipe

1. Cut the eggs and avocado into pieces and add to a bowl.

2. Mix with the lemon juice, mayonnaise, herbs, salt and pepper to the bowl and mix gently.

3. Place one fourth of the mixture onto each leaf and enjoy.

4. You can sprinkle on spices and finely chopped herbs to taste.

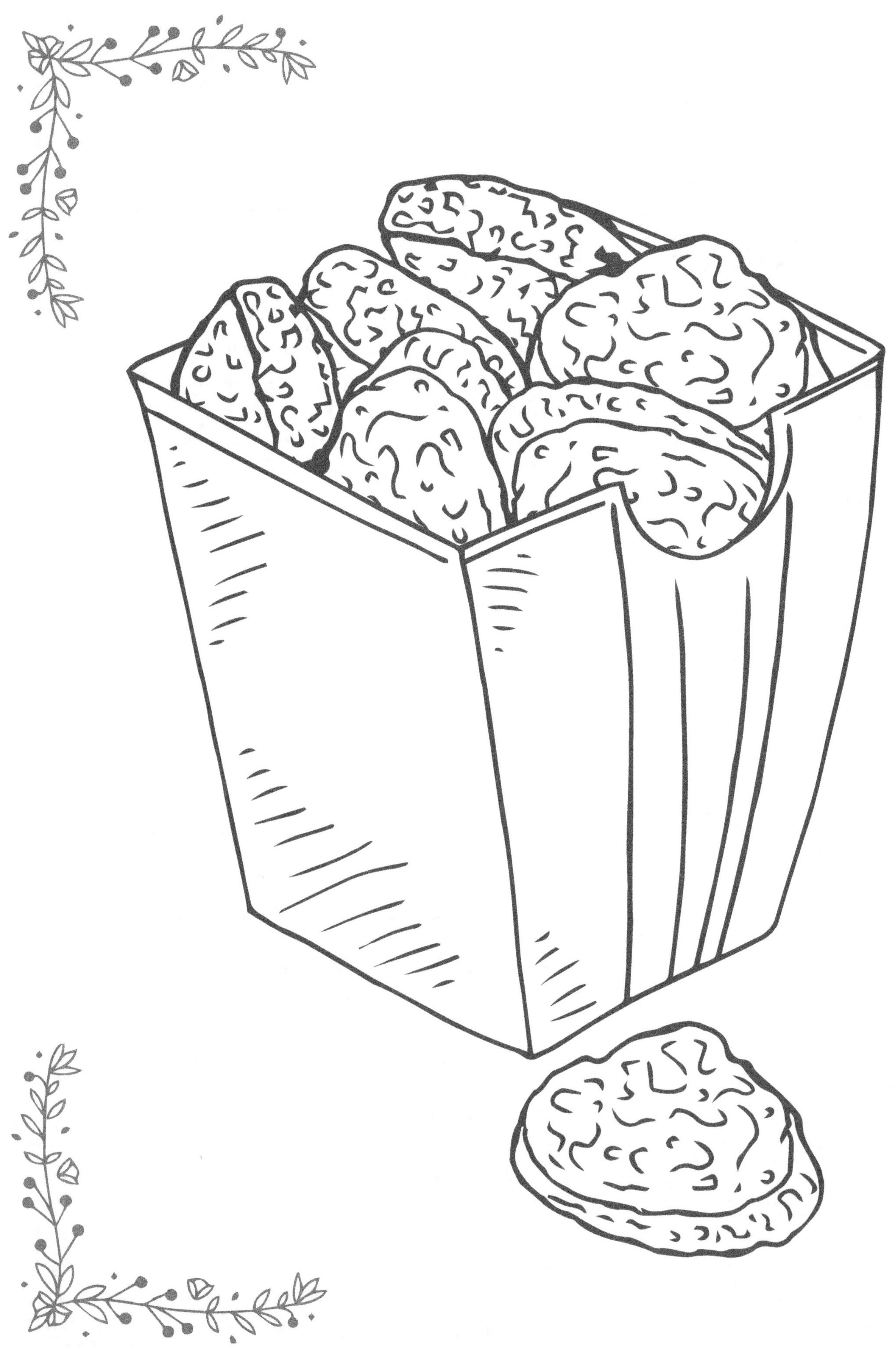

CHICKEN NUGGETS

<table>
<tr><td>Servings: 6</td></tr>
</table>

Nutritional Values Per Serving:

Net Carbs:	2 g	Protein:	18 g
Fat:	17 g	Calories:	243 kcal

Ingredients

2 boneless, skinless chicken breast halves

1 cup cream cheese

1 egg

¼ cup almond flour

1 tsp garlic

This is how you make the recipe

1. Preheat the oven to 350˚F.

2. Put the chicken in a food processor, add in the rest of the ingredients and mix until combined.

3. Spoon out scoops onto parchment-lined baking sheet

4. Bake for 12-14 minutes, until slightly golden and firm.

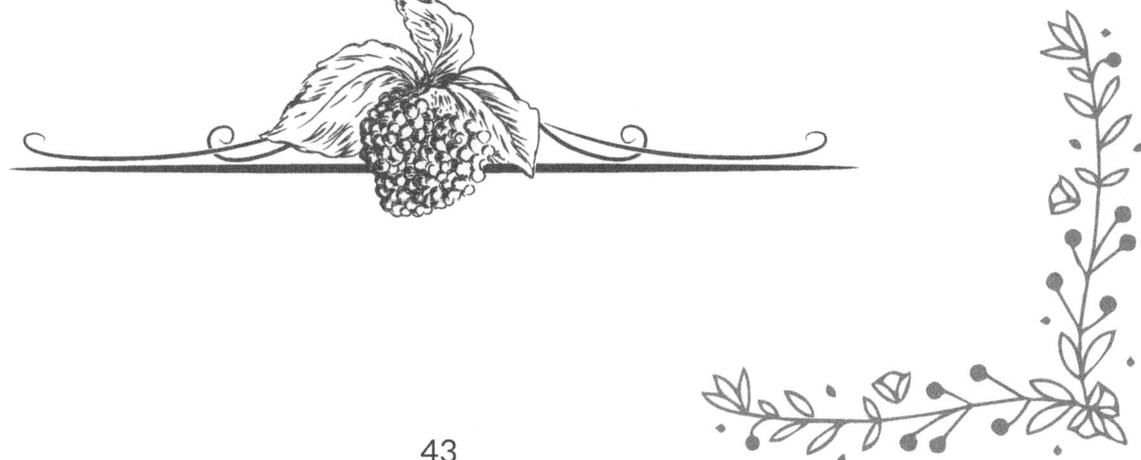

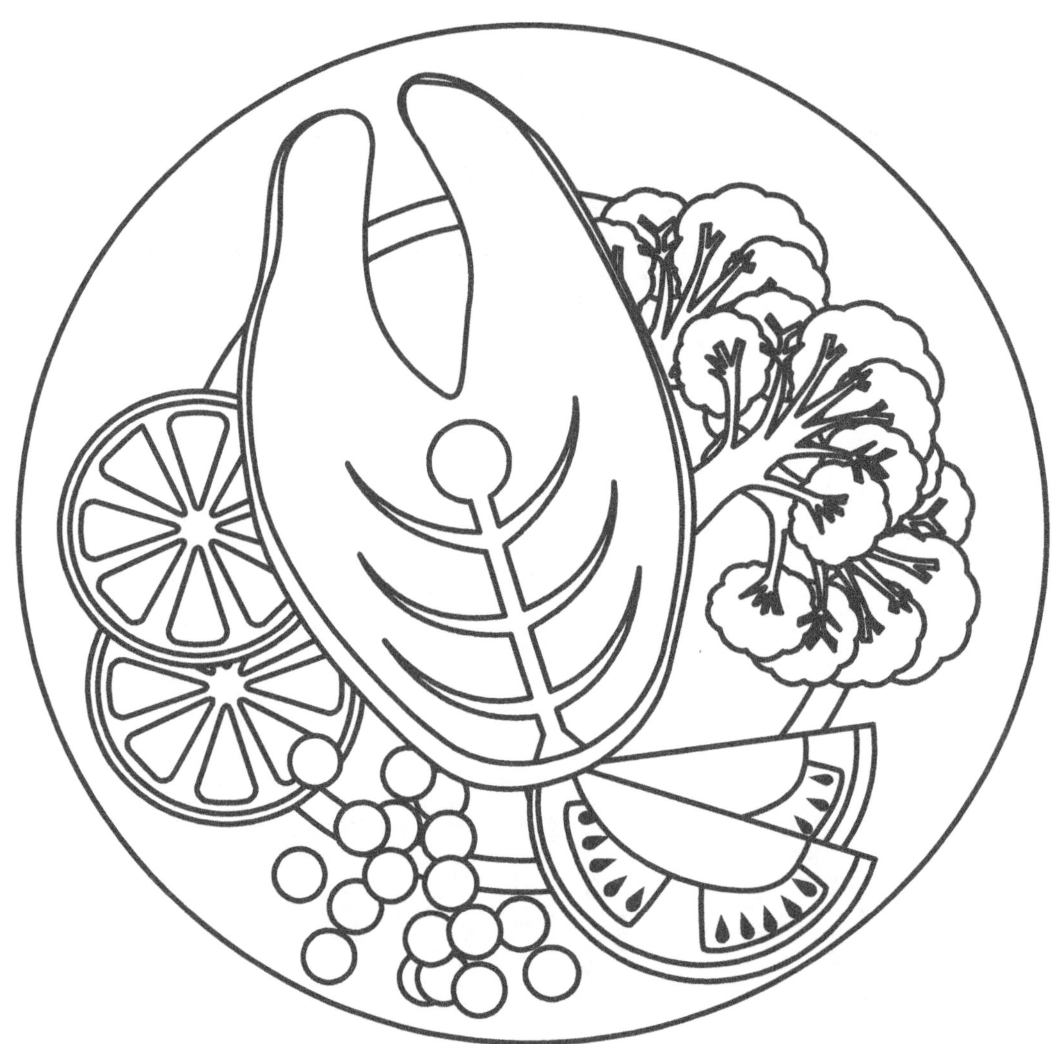

SALMON SALAD IN A JAR

Servings: 6

Nutritional Values Per Serving:
Net Carbs:	4 g	Protein:	71 g
Fat:	55 g	Calories:	799 kcal

Ingredients

3 large packages smoked salmon, chopped
2 cups leafy greens, cabbage/broccoli, roughly chopped
1½ cups cherry tomatoes, chopped
1 cup red peppers, sliced
1 cup cucumber, sliced

This is how you make the recipe

1. Wash and chop the vegetables.
2. Put the greens, cabbage or broccoli at the bottom of each jar.
3. Add sliced cucumbers, red peppers and tomatoes.
4. Top it off with pieces of salmon.
5. Just before serving, add a generous amount of dressing of your choice.

SAVORY SALMON FAT BOMBS

Servings: 6

Nutritional Values Per Serving:
Net Carbs:	0.7 g	Protein:	3.2 g
Fat:	15.7 g	Calories:	147 kcal

Ingredients

½ cup cream cheese
⅓ cup butter
½ package smoked salmon
1 tbsp lemon juice
1-2 tbsp dill

This is how you make the recipe

1. Mix the cream cheese, butter and smoked salmon.
2. Add lemon juice and dill and pulse until smooth.
3. Form small fat bombs using about 2½ tbsp of the mixture per piece.
4. Garnish with dill and place in the fridge for 1-2 hours.

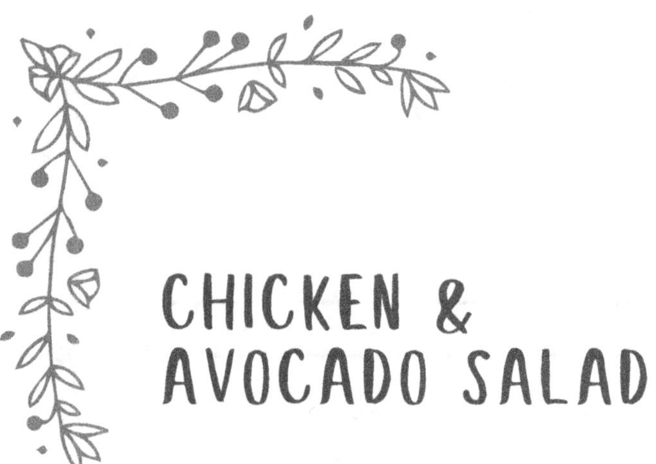

CHICKEN & AVOCADO SALAD

Servings: 4

Nutritional Values Per Serving:

Net Carbs:	6 g	Protein:	28 g
Fat:	34 g	Calories:	449 kcal

Ingredients

4 chicken breasts

5 romaine lettuce leaves

3 tomatoes, sliced

2 avocados, sliced

4 tbsp of pesto

This is how you make the recipe

1. Coat the chicken fillets with half of the pesto. Let marinade for 20 minutes.

2. Cook the chicken in a bit of avocado oil until each side is golden and fully cooked. Then slice the chicken into strips.

3. Prepare the salad with the romaine leaves, tomatoes and avocado slices.

4. Drizzle with remaining pesto and serve.

MARINATED STEAK SALAD

Servings: 2

Nutritional Values Per Serving:

Net Carbs:	2 g	Protein:	33 g
Fat:	37 g	Calories:	500 kcal

Ingredients

2 steaks

2 cups salad greens

½ red bell pepper

8 cherry tomatoes

¼ cup tamari soy sauce

Optional: 4 radishes

This is how you make the recipe

1. Have the steak soak in the Tamari Soy Sauce for half an hour.

2. Wash the salad greens and cut the bell pepper, tomatoes and radishes (optional).

3. Cook the steaks, salt them to taste, cut them into slices and place them on top of the salad greens. For additional flavour, add a little lemon juice and enjoy!

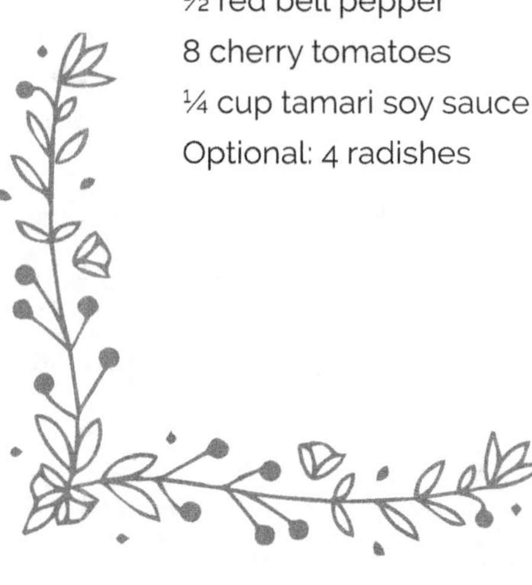

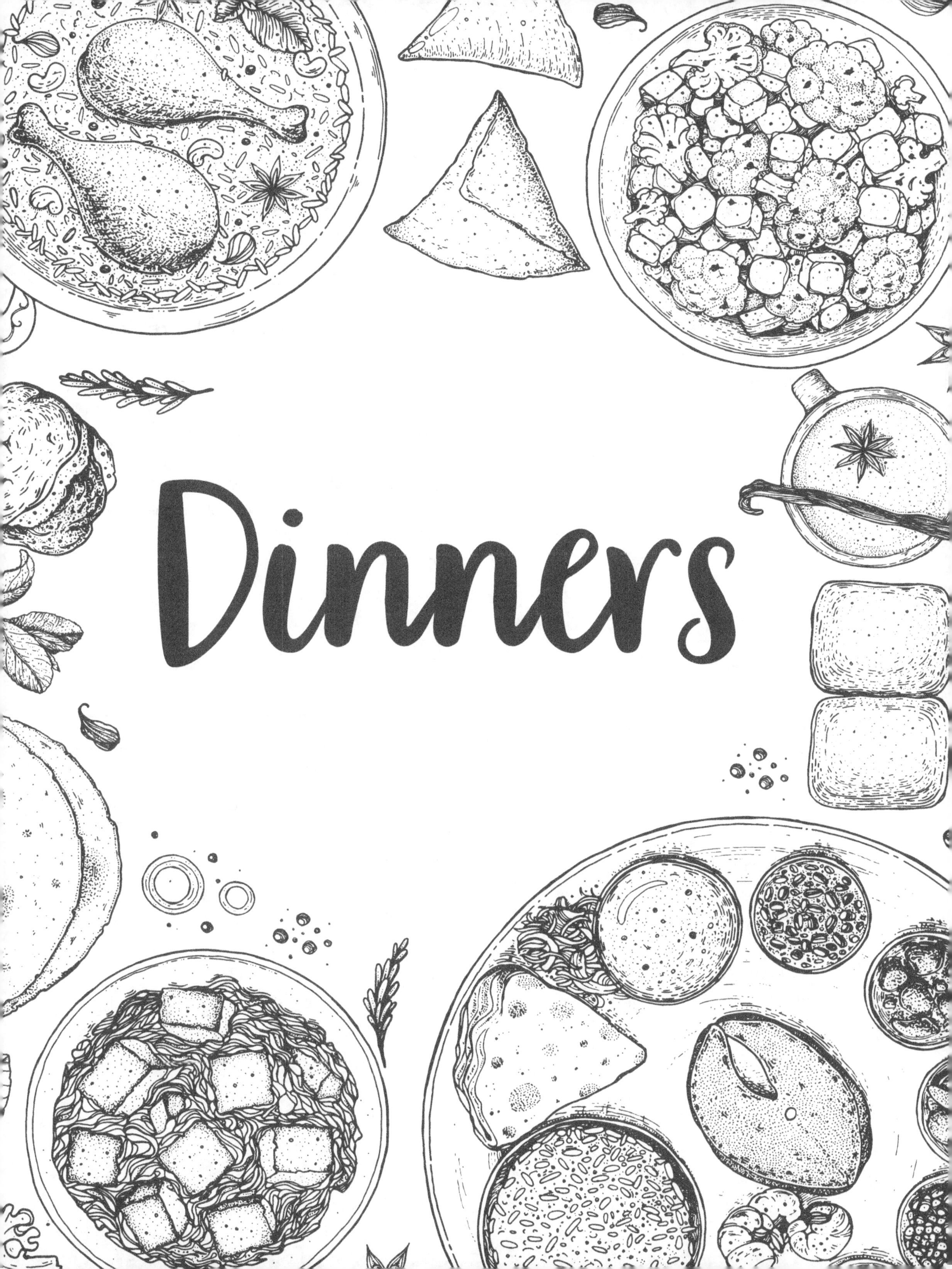

Dinners

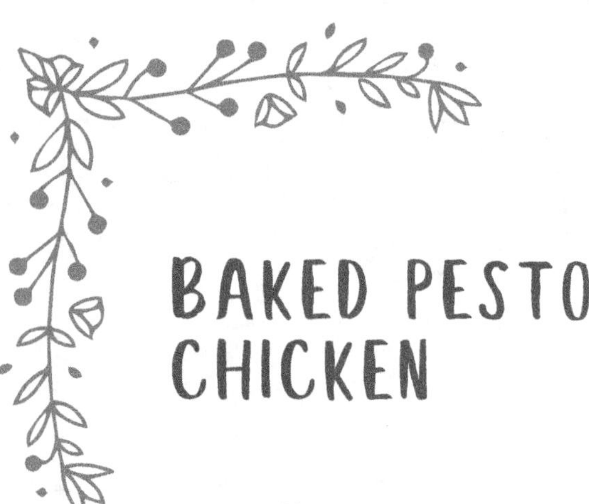

BAKED PESTO CHICKEN

Servings: 4

Nutritional Values Per Serving:

Net Carbs:	2 g	Protein:	61 g
Fat:	22 g	Calories:	471 kcal

Ingredients

4 chicken breasts

3 tbsp basil pesto

1 cup mozzarella, shredded

This is how you make the recipe

1. Preheat the oven to 350°F.

2. Slice each chicken breast in half to make eight pieces. Place them in an oiled baking dish and sprinkle with salt and pepper to taste.

3. Spread pesto onto the chicken pieces and then sprinkle the shredded mozzarella on top.

4. Bake for 35-45 minutes until the chicken is cooked and the cheese is golden.

5. Serve and enjoy!

CHICKEN & CHEESE

Servings: 6

Nutritional Values Per Serving:

Net Carbs:	3 g	Protein:	52 g
Fat:	23 g	Calories:	446 kcal

Ingredients

6 chicken breasts, cut into pieces

½ cup Parmesan cheese

2 cups mozzarella, sliced

1 cup spinach

Pinch of nutmeg and pepper

This is how you make the recipe

1. Preheat the oven to 400°F. Brush a baking dish with oil and add the spinach, nutmeg and chicken.

2. Top with Parmesan cheese, slices of mozzarella and pepper.

3. Bake for 35 minutes, until chicken is cooked.

LASAGNA STUFFED PEPPERS

Servings: 4

Nutritional Values Per Serving:
Net Carbs:	6.5 g	Protein:	32 g
Fat:	14 g	Calories:	281 kcal

Ingredients

4 large red bell peppers

2 tsp garlic, minced

1½ cups minced turkey

1½ cups ricotta cheese

2 cups mozzarella cheese

This is how you make the recipe

1. Preheat the oven to 400°F.

2. Cut off the tops of the red peppers and set aside. discard the seeds and insides.

3. Put the halved peppers on a oiled baking dish. Sprinkle with ¼ tsp garlic.

4. Portion out the turkey into each of the peppers. Sprinkle with more garlic and salt. Bake for 30 minutes.

5. Divide the ricotta cheese amongst the peppers and sprinkle the mozzarella on top.

6. If you wish, you could place cherry tomatoes around the peppers.

7. Bake for an additional 30 minutes until the peppers are softened and the cheese is golden.

COCONUT-LIME STEAK

Servings: 4

Nutritional Values Per Serving:
Net Carbs:	5 g	Protein:	35 g
Fat:	54 g	Calories:	661 kcal

Ingredients

4 steaks

Zest & juice from one lime

1 tbsp garlic, minced

1 tsp ginger, grated

½ cup coconut oil

This is how you make the recipe

1. In a bowl, combine the coconut oil, lime juice and zest, garlic and ginger. Add salt and crushed red pepper to taste.

2. Add the steak and let it marinate for 20 minutes.

3. Transfer steak to a pan and cook over medium-high heat.

4. Spoon the rest of the marinade out into the pan to cook with the steak.

5. Flip the steak and cook on both sides until it's cooked well, 4-5 minutes per side.

6. Serve and enjoy!

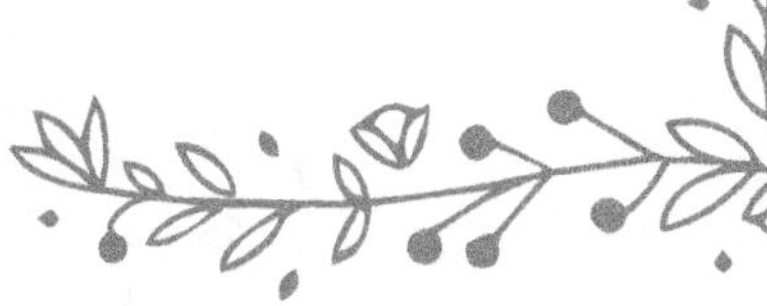

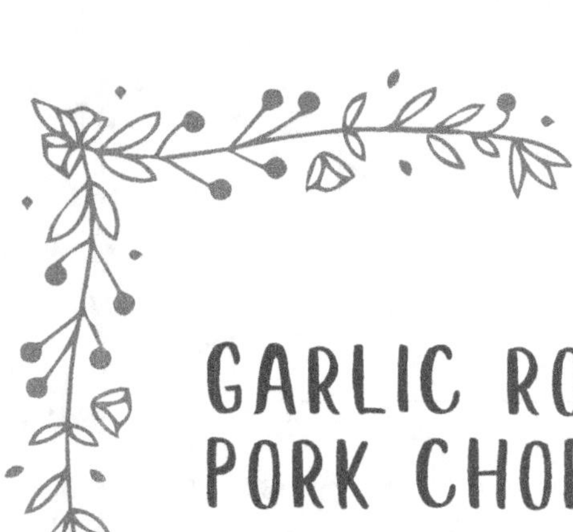

GARLIC ROSEMARY PORK CHOPS

Ingredients

4 pork loin chops
Rosemary, finely minced
1 clove garlic, minced
½ cup butter, softened
1 tbsp avocado oil

This is how you make the recipe

1. Preheat the oven to 375°F. Season chops with salt and pepper to taste.

2. Mix the butter, minced rosemary and garlic.

3. Place the chops in an oiled baking dish, place in the oven and cook the chops until golden, about 5 minutes, flip and cook 5 additional minutes.

4. Let the oven cool to 60°C.

5. Brush the herb butter over the chops and continue cooking for 15 more minutes.

BRUSSELS SPROUTS WITH BACON

Ingredients

16 slices of bacon
48 Brussels sprouts
Pinch salt and pepper
Mayonnaise

This is how you make the recipe

1. Preheat the oven to 400°F. Line baking sheet with parchment paper.

2. Clean and halve the brussels sprouts.

3. Cut bacon into small pieces.

4. Season the sprouts with salt and pepper, then bake together with the bacon for 35-40 minutes.

5. Serve with mayonnaise.

ITALIAN MEATBALLS

Yield: 8 meatballs

Nutritional Values Per Meatball:

Net Carbs:	0.7 g	Protein:	12.2 g
Fat:	10.9 g	Calories:	153 kcal

Ingredients

1 package of minced beef

1 egg

½ cup Parmesan, shredded

½ cup mozzarella. shredded

1 tbsp garlic, minced

This is how you make the recipe

1. Preheat the oven to 400°F. Line a baking tray with parchment paper.

2. In a bowl, combine all ingredients and knead together until combined.

3. Form into meatballs and place them on the baking tray.

4. Bake for 20 minutes and serve warm with herb-spiced cream.

ASPARAGUS & BACON CHICKEN

Servings: 4

Nutritional Values Per Serving:

Net Carbs:	2 g	Protein:	32 g
Fat:	25 g	Calories:	377 kcal

Ingredients

8 chicken tenders

8 slices of bacon

12 asparagus spears

4 small branches of rosemary

This is how you make the recipe

1. Preheat the oven to 400°F.

2. Lay two chicken tenders on top of each two pieces of bacon on a baking sheet. Sprinkle salt and pepper on them to taste.

3. Place three asparagus spears on top of each and then wrap the bacon around the chicken and asparagus to hold it all together.

4. Lay branches of rosemary on top for aroma.

5. Bake for 40 minutes.

6. Discard the rosemary and serve.

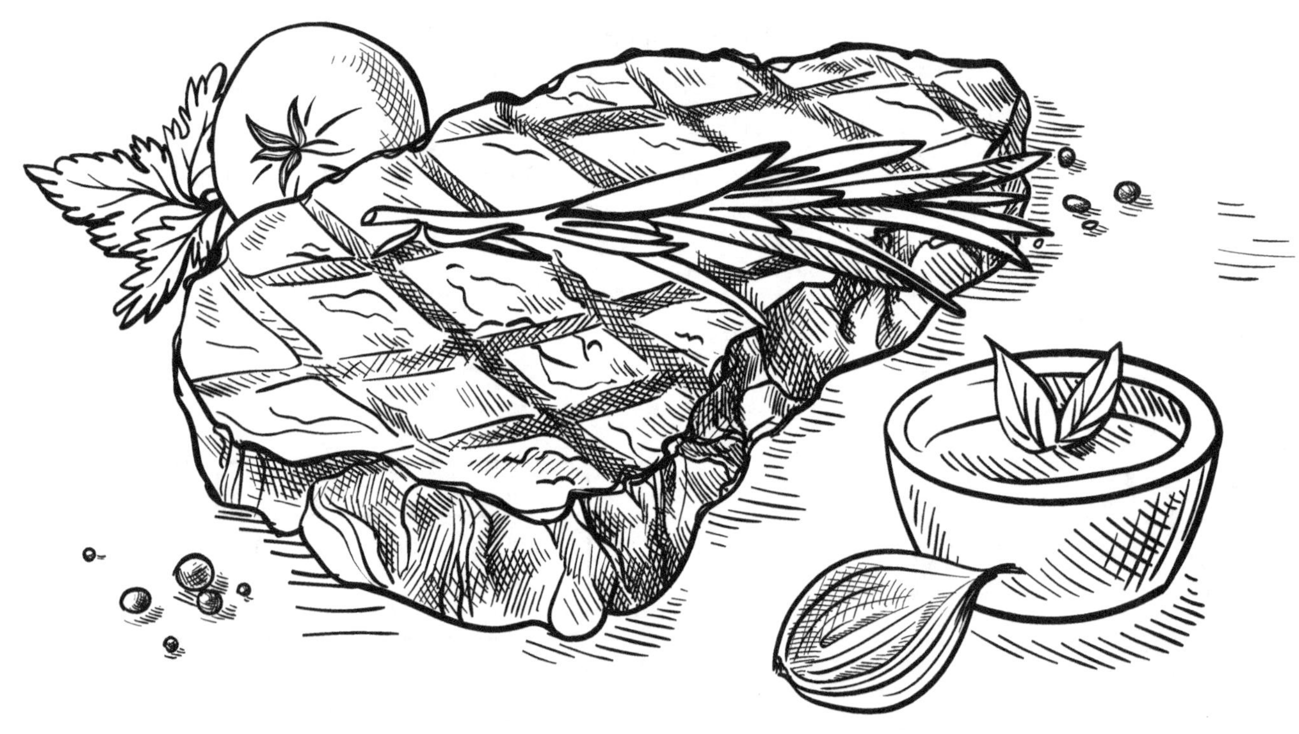

PEPPER STEAKS

Ingredients

4 boneless top loin steaks

2 tsp black pepper

¼ rosemary

1 tsp onion

1 tsp garlic

This is how you make the recipe

1. Chop the onion, mince the garlic and rosemary and place them in a bowl. Add pepper to taste.

2. Rub the mixture onto the steaks.

3. Coat a pan with oil and lay the steaks into it.

4. Cover them with a lid and cook over medium heat until the meat is done on both sides.

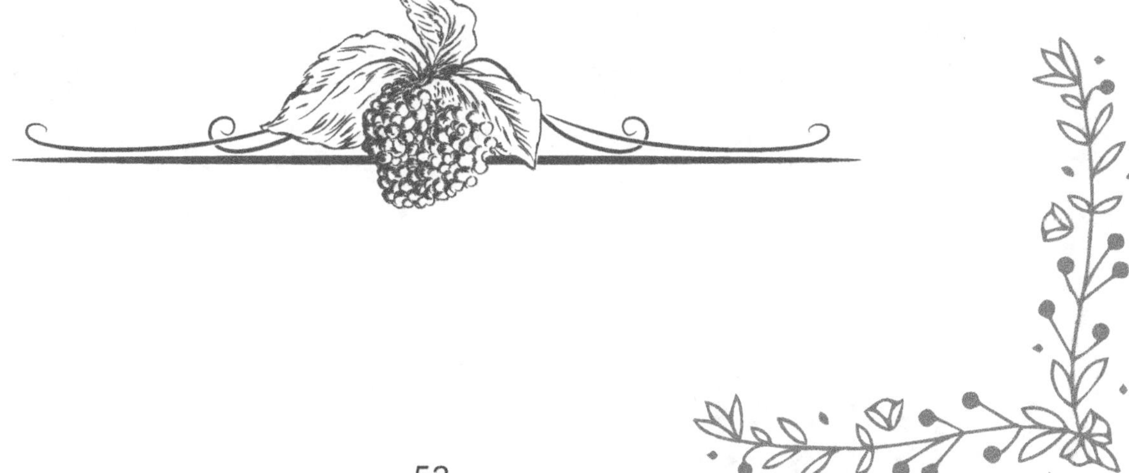

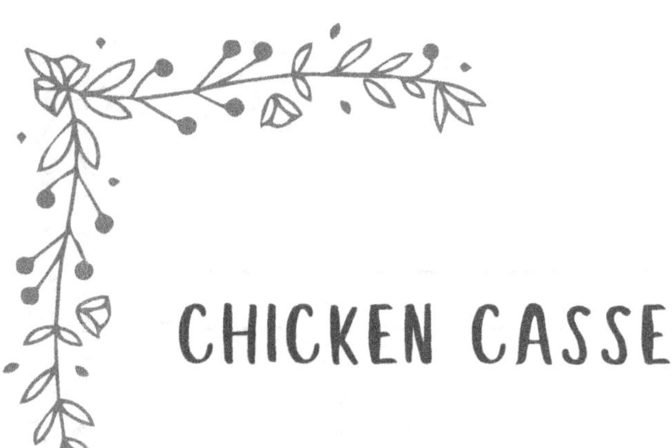

CHICKEN CASSEROLE

Servings: 8

Nutritional Values Per Serving:
Net Carbs: 3 g   Protein: 38 g
Fat: 30 g   Calories: 451 kcal

Ingredients

8 chicken breasts, cubed
¼ cup pesto
1 cup cream cheese
½ cup heavy cream
1 lb. mozzarella cheese

This is how you make the recipe

1. Preheat the oven to 400°F.
2. Mix the cream, pesto and cream cheese together until you have a smooth paste.
3. Cube half the mozzarella and add it with the chicken to the paste.
4. Place all in an oiled baking dish.
5. Shred the other half of the mozzarella and sprinkle it on top.
6. Bake for 30 minutes.
7. Tip: Serve with mashed cauliflower. Enjoy!

BASIL CHEESE CHICKEN

Servings: 2

Nutritional Values Per Serving:
Net Carbs: 1 g   Protein: 45 g
Fat: 25 g   Calories: 400 kcal

Ingredients

2 chicken breasts, with bone and skin
4 leaves of basil, chopped
2 tbsp cream cheese
2 tbsp mozzarella cheese, shredded
¼ tsp garlic, minced

This is how you make the recipe

1. Preheat the oven to 375°F.
2. Combine the cream cheese, garlic, basil and mozzarella. Salt and pepper to taste.
3. Insert the cheese stuffing under the skin of each breast.
4. Bake for 45 minutes.
5. Serve and enjoy!

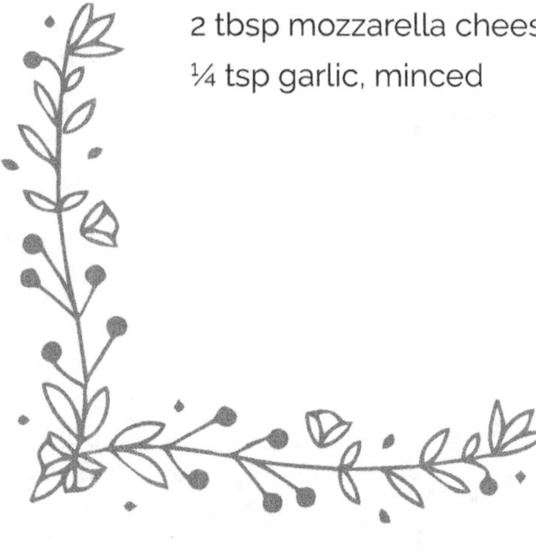

PESTO CHICKEN

Servings: 8

Nutritional Values Per Serving:
Net Carbs:	2 g	Protein:	21 g
Fat:	49 g	Calories:	550 kcal

Ingredients

16 boneless chicken thighs

1 cup cream cheese

1 cup mozzarella cheese, shredded

¼ cup basil pesto

¼ cup heavy cream

This is how you make the recipe

1. Preheat the oven to 400°F.

2. Place the thighs in the baking dish and bake for half an hour.

3. Combine the cream cheese, cream and pesto. Salt and pepper to taste.

4. Brush the sauce over the thighs, then sprinkle generously with mozzarella.

5. Bake for another 10 minutes, then serve.

PORK MEDALLIONS

Servings: 2

Nutritional Values Per Serving:
Net Carbs:	7 g	Protein:	46 g
Fat:	36 g	Calories:	519 kcal

Ingredients

2 pork tenderloins

3 medium shallots, minced

4 tbsp avocado oil

This is how you make the recipe

1. Slice the tenderloins into half-inch thick strips.

2. Coat each strip of pork with the minced shallots.

3. Cook the strips in avocado oil until done.

4. Serve with a nice fresh salad.

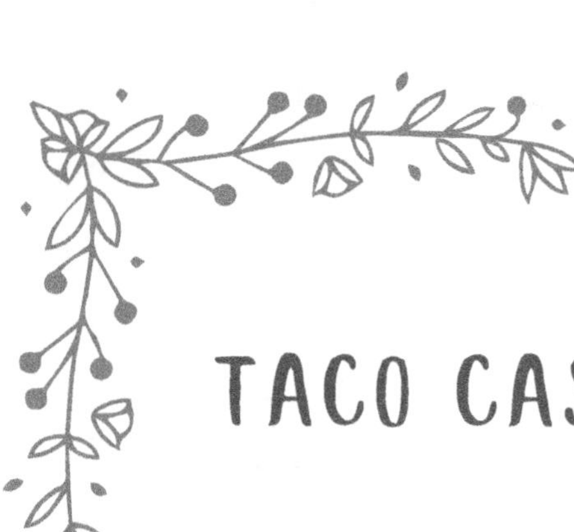

TACO CASSEROLE

<table><tr><td>Servings: 6</td></tr></table>

Servings: 6

Nutritional Values Per Serving:
Net Carbs: 6 g   Protein: 45 g
Fat: 18 g   Calories: 367 kcal

Ingredients

4 cups ground beef

2 cups cottage cheese

1 cup Cheddar cheese, shredded

1 cup salsa

2 tbsp taco seasoning

This is how you make the recipe

1. Preheat the oven to 400°F.

2. Mix the minced beef and taco seasoning in an 11x13-inch baking dish. Bake for 20 minutes.

3. Mix the cottage cheese, salsa, and half of the shredded Cheddar. Set aside.

4. Take the meat from the oven and drain the liquid out.

5. Stir the minced beef to make it crumbly. Spread the cheese and salsa on top.

6. Sprinkle the remaining Cheddar over the top.

7. Put the casserole back in the oven to bake for 20 more minutes.

PORK CHOPS

Servings: 6

Nutritional Values Per Serving:
Net Carbs: 2 g   Protein: 47 g
Fat: 25 g   Calories: 436 kcal

Ingredients

12 thin cut boneless pork CHOPS

4 cloves garlic

2 cups spinach

12 slices Cheddar or Swiss cheese

Herb mixture of your choice

This is how you make the recipe

1. Preheat the oven to 350°F.

2. Mince the garlic, add herbs, salt and pepper to taste and mix.

3. Spread this mixture on one side of the pork chops.

4. Lay 6 of the chops into a baking dish with the mixture side down.

5. Lay spinach leaves across the tops of these six chops .

6. Lay half of the cheese slices on top of the spinach layer.

7. Place the remaining chops on top of the first layer. With the garlic herb mixture side up.

8. Bake for 20 minutes.

9. Lay the remaining cheese slices on top of the chops and bake for an additional 12 minutes.

EASY SPICY CHICKEN

Servings: 3

Nutritional Values Per Serving:
Net Carbs: 3 g   Protein: 34 g
Fat: 17 g   Calories: 291 kcal

Ingredients

cream cheese

½ cup salsa

3 boneless, skinless chicken breast halves

1 tsp parsley, chopped

This is how you make the recipe

1. Preheat the oven to 350°F.

2. Cut the cream cheese into large chunks, then place them in a saucepan with the salsa, Salt and pepper to taste. Cook on the stove until it all combines.

3. Lay the chicken breasts in a baking dish and pour the cream cheese sauce over them.

4. Bake for 40-45 minutes.

5. Sprinkle with parsley and serve.

RANCH CHICKEN

Servings: 6

Nutritional Values Per Serving:
Net Carbs: 2 g   Protein: 54 g
Fat: 3 g   Calories: 257 kcal

Ingredients

12 chicken tenders

⅓ cup plain yogurt

1 tbsp dill

1 tbsp onion

1 tbsp garlic

This is how you make the recipe

1. Preheat the oven to 400°F.

2. Finely dice the dill, onion and garlic.

3. Mix with the yogurt in a bowl. Salt to taste.

4. Wash and dry the chicken tenders and add them to the marinade.

5. Let marinade for 3 hours.

6. Bake for 25-30 minutes until the chicken is cooked through.

7. If you wish, sprinkle parsley on top before cooking.

8. Serve and enjoy!

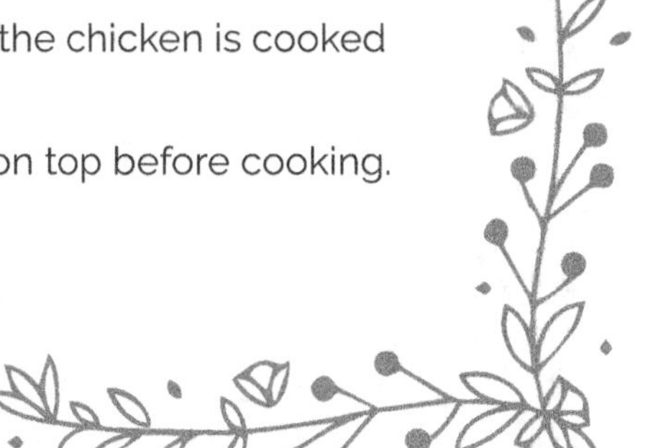

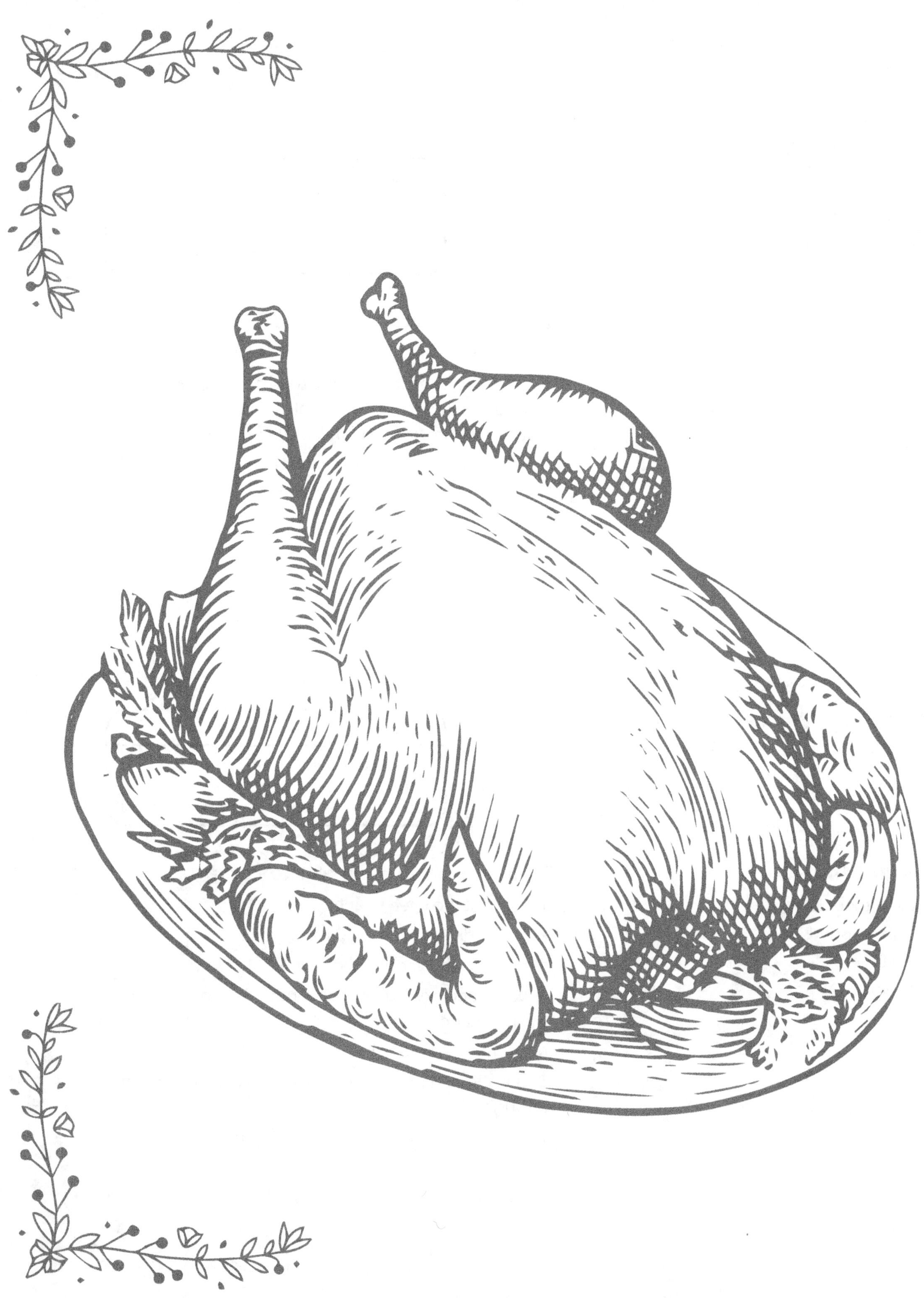

ROSEMARY ROAST CHICKEN

<table>
<tr><td colspan="2">Servings: 6</td></tr>
<tr><td colspan="2">Nutritional Values Per Serving:</td></tr>
<tr><td>Net Carbs: 0 g</td><td>Protein: 44 g</td></tr>
<tr><td>Fat: 24 g</td><td>Calories: 405 kcal</td></tr>
</table>

Ingredients

1 whole chicken

2 tsp olive oil

1 tsp thyme

1 tsp rosemary, minced

This is how you make the recipe

1. Rub the outside of chicken with salt and pepper. Refrigerate overnight.

2. Preheat the oven to 450°F.

3. Place the chicken, breast side up, in a baking dish and place in the oven.

4. After 15 minutes, brush it with oil, sprinkle on the herbs and continue roasting for another 40 minutes.

5. Remove the chicken from the oven and let it stand for 10 minutes before carving and serving.

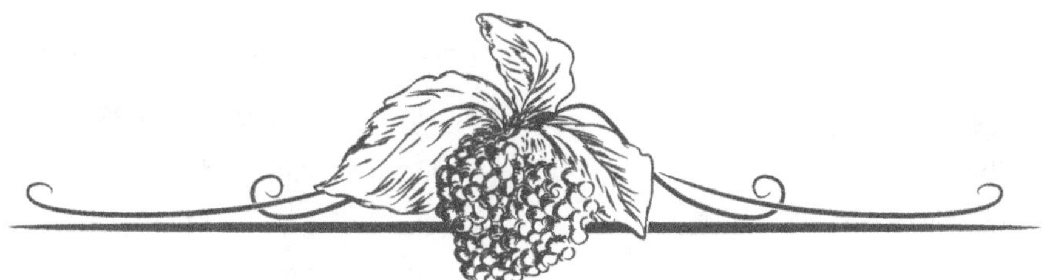

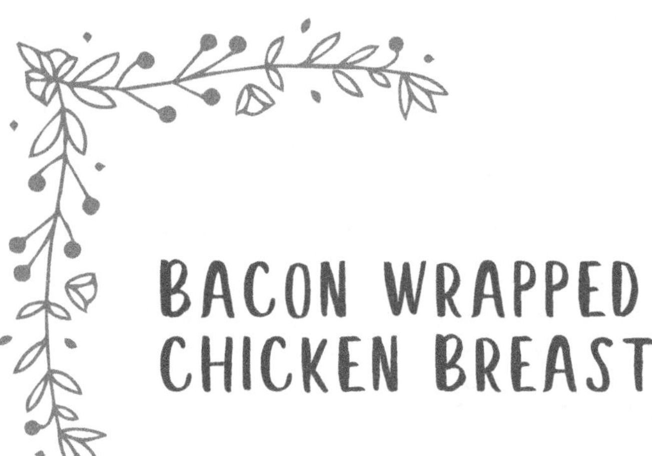

BACON WRAPPED CHICKEN BREAST

Ingredients

6 chicken breasts

2 tbsp seasoned salt (salt, pepper, garlic, onion and paprika powders)

6 slices of bacon

½ cup Cheddar cheese, shredded

Mustard or barbecue sauce

This is how you make the recipe

1. Preheat the oven to 400°F. Brush oil or butter on a baking sheet.

2. Cut each breast and each slice of bacon in half lengthwise.

3. Rub the seasoning on the chicken pieces, then wrap each piece with a slice of bacon.

4. Bake for 30 minutes until the chicken is cooked and the bacon is crispy.

5. Remove from the oven and sprinkle the Cheddar on top. Bake for an additional ten minutes until the cheese is golden.

6. Serve with mustard or barbecue sauce.

BAKED CHICKEN

Ingredients

4 chicken breasts

3 tbsp basil pesto

1 cup mozzarella, thinly sliced

This is how you make the recipe

1. Preheat the oven to 350°F.

2. Coat a baking dish with oil or butter.

3. Cut the chicken breasts in half and place them in the dish. Spread the pesto on the chicken and salt and pepper to taste.

4. Lay slices of the mozzarella on top.

5. Bake for 35-45 minutes until the chicken is well cooked and the cheese is golden and bubbly.

MARINARA CHICKEN CASSEROLE

Servings: 6

Nutritional Values Per Serving:

Net Carbs:	4 g	Protein:	35 g
Fat:	24 g	Calories:	383 kcal

Ingredients

6 chicken breasts

1 cup cream cheese

1 tsp garlic, minced

1 cup marinara sauce

1 cup mozzarella, shredded

This is how you make the recipe

1. Preheat the oven to 350°F.

2. Cut chicken into small pieces, coat a baking dish with oil and lay in the chicken.

3. Mix the cream cheese and garlic, then salt and pepper to taste.

4. Spread the sauce onto the chicken, sprinkle with mozzarella and bake for 30 minutes.

PIZZA CASSEROLE

Servings: 6

Nutritional Values Per Serving:

Net Carbs:	7 g	Protein:	14 g
Fat:	16 g	Calories:	238 kcal

Ingredients

1 head of cauliflower

2 cups mozzarella cheese, shredded

1½ cups marinara sauce

24 slices of pepperoni

2 tsp Italian seasoning

This is how you make the recipe

1. Preheat the oven to 425°F.

2. Cut the cauliflower into small florets, then place in an oiled baking dish.

3. Sprinkle with olive oil, salt and pepper.

4. Bake for 25 minutes.

5. Remove from the oven and pour the marinara sauce over the cauliflower.

6. Sprinkle the mozzarella onto the cauliflower and top it with Italian seasoning.

7. Lay the pepperoni or salami slices onto the cheese.

8. Return the casserole to the oven to bake for 10 more minutes.

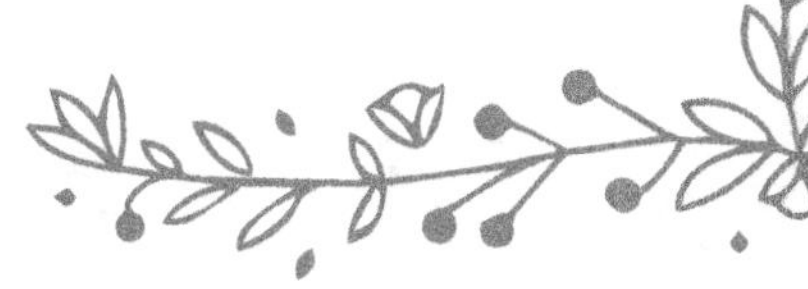

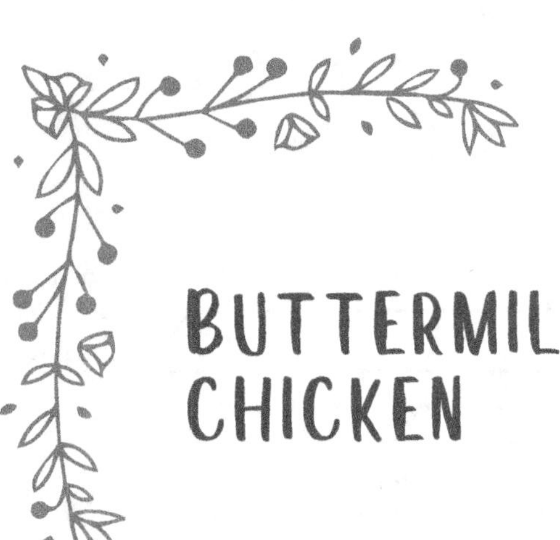

BUTTERMILK CHICKEN

Servings: 12

Nutritional Values Per Serving:
Net Carbs:	1 g	Protein:	35 g
Fat:	4 g	Calories:	189 kcal

Ingredients

12 boneless, skinless chicken breast halves
1½ cups buttermilk
4 thyme
4 cloves garlic

This is how you make the recipe

1. Place the buttermilk, thyme, garlic in a bowl. Salt to taste.

2. Lay in the chicken and let marinate for 3 hours.

3. Preheat the oven to 400°F.

4. Pour out and dispose of the marinade.

5. Cover the chicken with foil in a baking dish and bake for 15-20 minutes.

MARINATED LOBSTER TAILS

Servings: 6   Serving size: 1 lobster tail

Nutritional Values Per Serving:
Net Carbs:	2 g	Protein:	43 g
Fat:	29 g	Calories:	446 kcal

Ingredients

6 lobster tails
3 tbsp chives, minced
3 cloves garlic, minced
¾ cup avocado oil

This is how you make the recipe

1. Loosen the meat from the shell but keep the fin attached. Lift the meat and lay over the shell.

2. In a bowl, combine the chives, garlic and oil and then spoon it over the lobster. Let it marinade for 20 minutes.

3. Place lobster tails, meat side up, on a pan and cover it with a lid.

4. Cook over medium heat for 10 minutes, until the meat is tender. Enjoy!

BUFFALO PULLED CHICKEN

Servings: 6			
Nutritional Values Per Serving:			
Net Carbs:	6 g	Protein:	23 g
Fat:	3 g	Calories:	147 kcal

Ingredients

4 boneless, skinless chicken breast halves

½ cup Buffalo wing sauce

2 tsp sour cream

2 tsp cup mayo

1 tsp mixed herbs (i.e. garlic, onion, parsley, dill, etc.)

This is how you make the recipe

1. Place all of the ingredients into a slow cooker, cover it and cook on low for 3-4 hours, until meat is tender.

2. Shred the chicken, cover with wing sauce and serve.

3. Tip: A tasty variety is to serve the chicken covered in shredded cheese.

ITALIAN PORK CHOPS

Servings: 4			
Nutritional Values Per Serving:			
Net Carbs:	2 g	Protein:	40 g
Fat:	20 g	Calories:	365 kcal

Ingredients

4 boneless pork loin chops

2½ cups broccoli

2 roasted red peppers, chopped

1 tsp garlic, minced

½ cup mozzarella cheese

This is how you make the recipe

1. Preheat the oven to 350°F.

2. Steam the broccoli for 7 minutes.

3. Sprinkle pork chops with the garlic and add salt and pepper to taste.

4. Lay the chops in a baking dish and cook for 20 minutes, until internal temperature reaches at least 145°F. Then remove from the oven.

5. Turn on the broiler.

6. Cover the chops with red peppers, broccoli and the cheese. Broil for 4 minutes. Serve and enjoy!

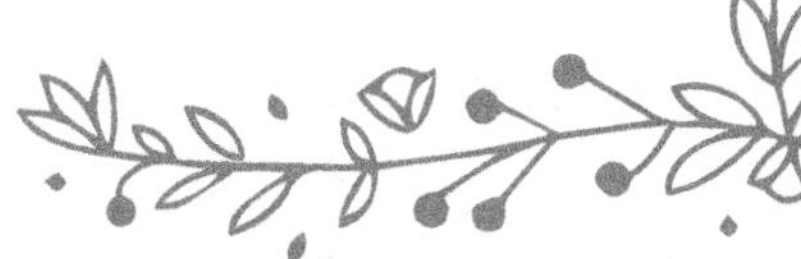

PISTACHIO SALMON

Ingredients

1 lb. salmon fillet

¼ cup Parmesan cheese, grated

⅓ cup pistachios, chopped

¼ cup breadcrumbs

1 tbsp lemon juice

This is how you make the recipe

1. Preheat the oven to 400°F.

2. In a bowl, mix the chopped pistachios with breadcrumbs and cheese.

3. Place the salmon in an oiled pan with the skin side down. Drizzle with the lemon juice and sprinkle on salt and pepper to taste.

4. Top with the pistachio mixture.

5. Bake, uncovered, for 15 minutes.

6. Lift the salmon from its skin, serve and enjoy!

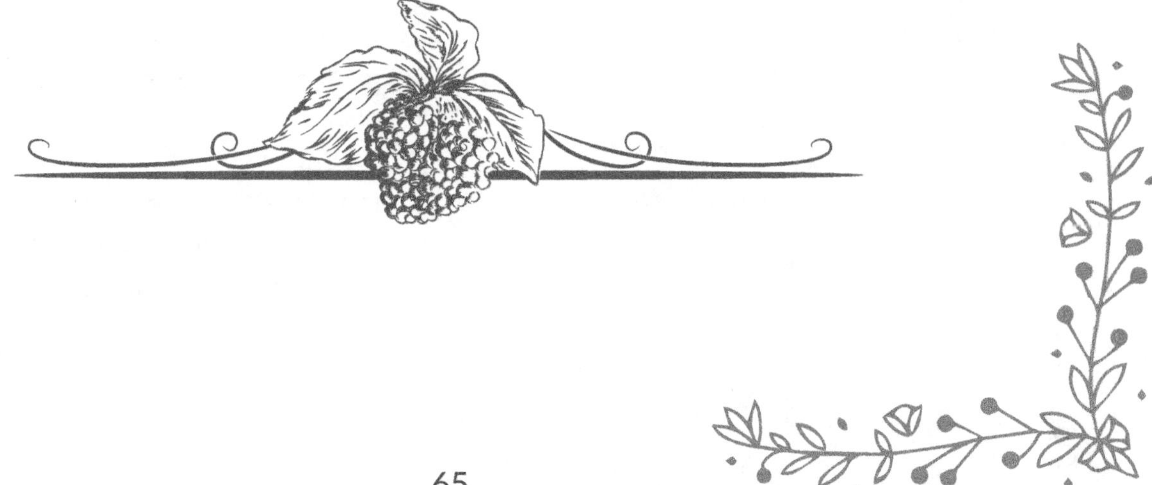

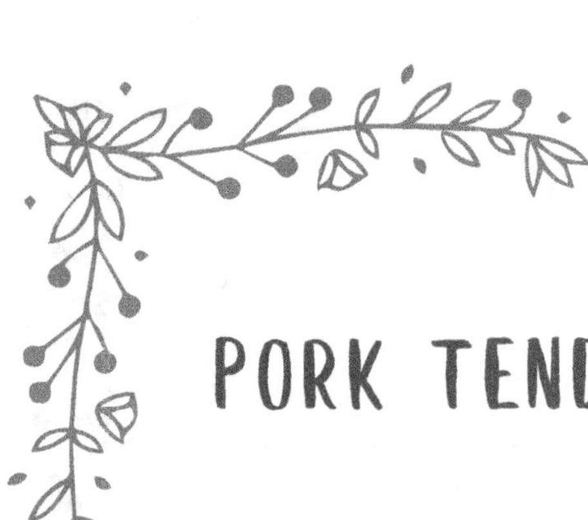

PORK TENDERLOIN

Ingredients

10 slices of bacon

1 pork tenderloin

⅓ cup pesto

1 cup Romano cheese, grated

1 cup baby spinach

This is how you make the recipe

1. Preheat the oven to 425˚F.

2. Lay the slices of bacon in a pan so they slightly overlap.

3. Make a lengthwise cut down the center of the tenderloin, cutting within ½-inch from the bottom. Open the tenderloin flat like an open-face sandwich and pound it with a meat mallet so that it is all ½-inch thick.

4. Place the tenderloin on top of the bacon, perpendicular to the slices. Sprinkle with salt and pepper to taste.

5. Spread pesto onto it and then sprinkle on the cheese and spinach.

6. Close the tenderloin, then wrap it with the bacon. Tie it with kitchen string every few inches.

7. Brown the fillet in the pan on both sides for 8 minutes.

8. Shift the loin to a baking dish and roast it in the oven for 20 minutes, until the inside temperature reaches at least 145˚.

9. Remove the string, let stand 5 minutes before slicing and serving.

COD & ASPARAGUS BAKE

Ingredients

4 cod fillets

2½ cups asparagus

2 cups cherry tomatoes, halved

2 tbsp lemon juice

¼ cup Romano or Parmesan cheese, grated

This is how you make the recipe

1. Preheat the oven to 375˚F.

2. Place the cod and asparagus in an oiled baking dish.

3. Brush the fish with lemon juice and add the tomatoes. Sprinkle the cheese on top. You can sprinkle on lemon zest as well to add more flavour.

4. Bake for 14 minutes, until done, then serve.

GARLIC CHICKEN WITH WINE

Servings: 4

Nutritional Values Per Serving:

Net Carbs:	4 g	Protein:	36 g
Fat:	7 g	Calories:	243 kcal

Ingredients

4 chicken breast halves

2 cups baby portabella mushrooms, sliced

1 onion, chopped

2 garlic cloves, minced

½ cup dry white wine

This is how you make the recipe

1. Pound the chicken breasts so that they become ½-inch thick. Sprinkle with salt and pepper to taste.

2. Cook the chicken in an oiled pan for 5-6 minutes per side.

3. Remove the chicken from the pan, then drop in the mushrooms and onions and cook them until browned.

4. Add garlic to the mushrooms and onion and stir for a moment.

5. Add the wine and stir until it boils, and the sauce is slightly reduced.

6. Pour it over the chicken and serve with vegetables.

CHICKEN BREASTS

Servings: 4

Nutritional Values Per Serving:

Net Carbs:	1 g	Protein:	40 g
Fat:	17 g	Calories:	332 kcal

Ingredients

4 chicken breast halves

1 cup crumbled feta cheese

⅓ cup oil-packed, sun-dried tomatoes, chopped

2 tbsp olive oil from sun-dried tomatoes, divided

1 tsp herb and spice mix - oregano, thyme, salt, pepper, paprika

This is how you make the recipe

1. Preheat the oven to 375°F. Mix cheese and chopped tomatoes.

2. Pound chicken breasts with a meat mallet to ¼-inch thickness.

3. Brush with 1 tbsp oil; sprinkle with seasoning mix. Sprinkle on the feta cheese.

4. Roll up the breast and secure with a toothpick.

5. Place the chicken in an oiled baking dish, brush oil and bake for 35 minutes.

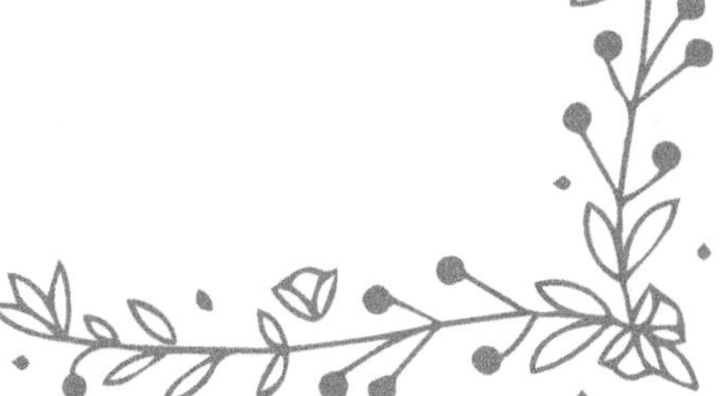

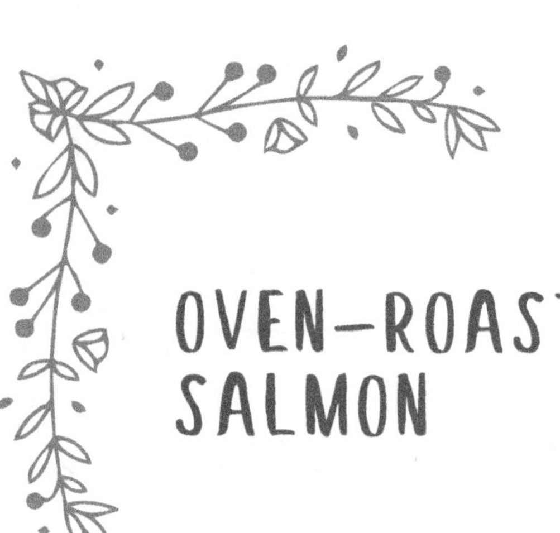

OVEN-ROASTED SALMON

Servings: 4

Nutritional Values Per Serving:
Net Carbs: 0 g   Protein: 29 g
Fat: 19 g   Calories: 295 kcal

Ingredients

1 large salmon fillet
1 tbsp olive oil
1 tbsp lemon juice
Herb mix: parsley, garlic, dill

This is how you make the recipe

1. Preheat the oven to 450°F.

2. Brush the salmon with oil and drizzle on the lemon juice, salt and pepper to taste.

3. Lay the salmon, skin side down in a baking dish. Bake for 14-18 minutes.

4. Serve and enjoy.

MUSHROOM-STUFFED CHICKEN

Servings: 4

Nutritional Values Per Serving:
Net Carbs: 4 g   Protein: 41 g
Fat: 25 g   Calories: 420 kcal

Ingredients

4 boneless skinless chicken breast halves
4 slices of bacon
1 shallot, finely chopped
¾ cup mushrooms, chopped
½ cup prepared pesto

This is how you make the recipe

1. Preheat the oven to 350°F

2. Partially cook the bacon, then dry it on a paper towel.

3. Cook the shallot for about 2 minutes, add the mushrooms and continue cooking for another 2 minutes. Add salt and pepper to taste.

4. Pound the chicken breasts until they are ¼-inch thick.

5. Brush on the pesto, lay the bacon on them and cover with the mushroom mixture.

6. Fold chicken in half, enclosing the mixture and secure them with toothpicks.

7. Place them in a baking dish and bake for half an hour, until the internal temperature reaches at least 165°F.

8. Serve and enjoy!

Side
Dishes

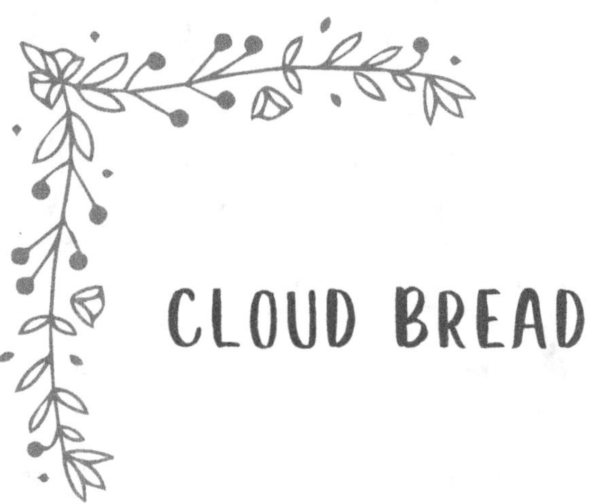

CLOUD BREAD

<table>
<tr><td>Yield: 20</td></tr>
</table>

Nutritional Values Per Serving:
Net Carbs: 0.4 g   Protein: 2.2 g
Fat: 2.8 g   Calories: 35 kcal

Ingredients

6 eggs
6 tbsp cream cheese
½ tsp cream of tartar
2 tsp herbs mix: rosemary, oregano,
basil, thyme

This is how you make the recipe

1. Preheat the oven to 300°F. . Line a baking tray t with   parchment paper.

2. Separate the egg and mix the yolk with the cream cheese and the herbs until well-combined.

3. Mix the egg whites with the cream of tartar or baking powder and a little salt until it forms stiff peaks.

4. Fold the two mixtures together.

5. Spoon portions onto the baking tray and bake for 30 minutes.

6. Enjoy with butter!

CAULIFLOWER MAC & CHEESE

Servings: 6   Serving size: ½ cup

Nutritional Values Per Serving:
Net Carbs: 6 g   Protein: 14 g
Fat: 33 g   Calories: 393 kcal

Ingredients

1 head of cauliflower, cut into small
florets
1 cup heavy cream
1 cup sharp Cheddar cheese, shredded
¼ cup cream cheese
1¼ tsp paprika

This is how you make the recipe

1. Preheat the oven to 375°F.

2. Steam the cauliflower for 4-5 minutes just until they just start to become tender. Pat dry.

3. Mix the cream, Cheddar, cream cheese and paprika. Salt and pepper to taste.

4. Place the mixture into a buttered baking dish.

5. Add the cauliflower and bake for 25 minutes.

CAULIFLOWER PIZZA CRUST

Servings: 8

Nutritional Values Per Serving:

Net Carbs:	3 g	Protein:	10 g
Fat:	6 g	Calories:	106 kcal

Ingredients

1 head of cauliflower, cut into florets

1½ cup Parmesan cheese, grated

1 egg

½ tbsp oregano & thyme mix

½ tsp garlic, minced

This is how you make the recipe

1. Preheat the oven to 400°F. Line a baking sheet or pizza pan with parchment paper.

2. Pulse the cauliflower in a food processor.

3. In a pan, stir fry the cauliflower for 10 minutes until very soft.

4. In a bowl, whisk the egg with the cheese, garlic and herbs.

5. When the cauliflower is soft, dump it onto a towel and squeeze out the water into the sink.

6. Mash the cauliflower with the cheese and egg mixture.

7. Press the pizza dough onto the baking tray to ¼ inch thickness.

8. Place in the oven and bake for 20 minutes, until the top is dry and firm.

9. Remove and let cool.

10. It's now ready for your added toppings.

BROCCOLI & CHEDDAR BREAD

Servings: 10

Nutritional Values Per Serving:

Net Carbs:	1 g	Protein:	6 g
Fat:	6 g	Calories:	90 kcal

Ingredients

5 eggs

1 cup cheddar cheese

¾ cup broccoli

3½ tbsp coconut flour

2 tsp baking powder

This is how you make the recipe

1. Preheat the oven to 350°F. Line a loaf dish with parchment paper.

2. Cut the broccoli into very small florets and shred the cheese.

3. In a bowl, whisk the eggs and then combine all of the ingredients.

4. Pour the mixture into the loaf dish and bake for 35 minutes.

5. Let it cool, then slice and enjoy!

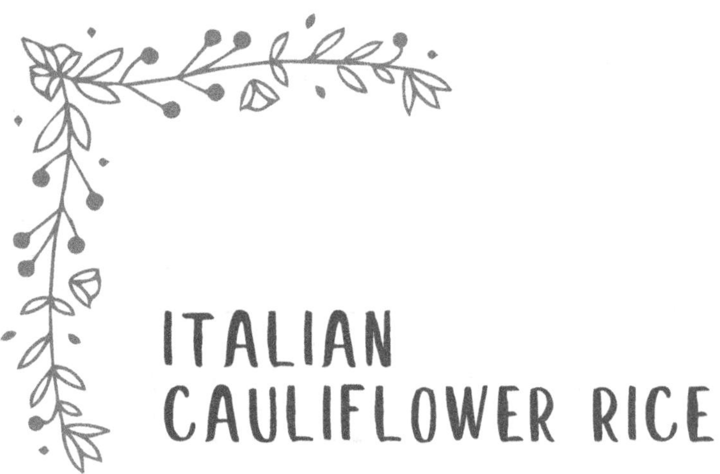

ITALIAN CAULIFLOWER RICE

<table>
<tr><td>Servings: 6</td><td></td><td></td><td></td></tr>
<tr><td colspan="4">Nutritional Values Per Serving:</td></tr>
<tr><td>Net Carbs:</td><td>3 g</td><td>Protein:</td><td>4 g</td></tr>
<tr><td>Fat:</td><td>9 g</td><td>Calories:</td><td>112 kcal</td></tr>
</table>

Ingredients

1 head of cauliflower
2 tbsp unsalted butter
1 tbsp olive oil
1½ tsp mix of garlic, thyme, rosemary, oregano
½ cup Asiago cheese

This is how you make the recipe

1. Grate the cauliflower into rice.

2. In a pan, heat the oil and butter. Add the garlic and herbs.

3. Stir in the cauliflower and cook uncovered for 15 minutes.

4. Stir in the cheese until well-combined.

5. Enjoy!

SPICY EDAMAME

<table>
<tr><td>Servings: 6</td><td></td><td></td><td></td></tr>
<tr><td colspan="4">Nutritional Values Per Serving:</td></tr>
<tr><td>Net Carbs:</td><td>3 g</td><td>Protein:</td><td>4 g</td></tr>
<tr><td>Fat:</td><td>2 g</td><td>Calories:</td><td>52 kcal</td></tr>
</table>

Ingredients

2 cups edamame
¾ tsp ginger, minced
½ tsp garlic, minced

This is how you make the recipe

1. Place the edamame in a pan and cover with water.

2. Cook for 4 minutes until it is soft.

3. Pour off the water, then mix with the ginger, garlic and red pepper. Salt to taste and enjoy!

CAULIFLOWER MASH

Servings: 6	Serving size: ⅔ cup

Nutritional Values Per Serving:

Net Carbs:	3 g	Protein:	2 g
Fat:	0 g	Calories:	26 kcal

Ingredients

1 head of cauliflower, chopped

½ cup chicken broth

2 cloves garlic

1 tsp whole peppercorns

1 bay leaf

This is how you make the recipe

1. Place the cauliflower in a steamer. Cover it and steam for 12 minutes. Drain in a colander.
2. Combine and boil the remaining ingredients in a saucepan.
3. Remove the peppercorns, garlic, and the bay leaf.
4. Blend the cauliflower until smooth and creamy.

PIMENTO CHEESE SPREAD

Yield: 1¼ cups	Serving size: 2 tbsp

Nutritional Values Per Serving:

Net Carbs:	1 g	Protein:	4 g
Fat:	11 g	Calories:	116 kcal

Ingredients

1½ cups Cheddar cheese, shredded

1 jar diced pimientos, drained and finely chopped

⅓ cup mayonnaise

This is how you make the recipe

1. Mix all of the ingredients together.
2. Enjoy as a dip or spread.

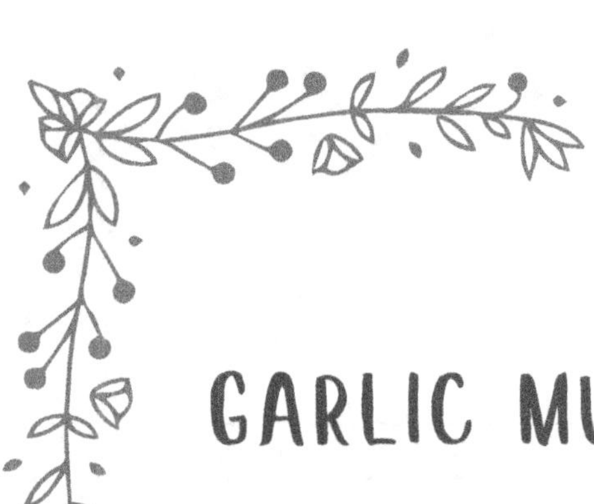

GARLIC MUSHROOMS

Ingredients

¾ lb champignon mushrooms

3 tsp garlic

1 tbsp breadcrumbs

⅓ cup butter, cubed

1 tbsp herb mix - thyme, sage, rosemary, oregano

This is how you make the recipe

1. Sauté the mushrooms with butter in a pan, add the garlic, herbs and breadcrumbs until mushrooms are tender. Salt and pepper to taste.

2. Serve and enjoy!

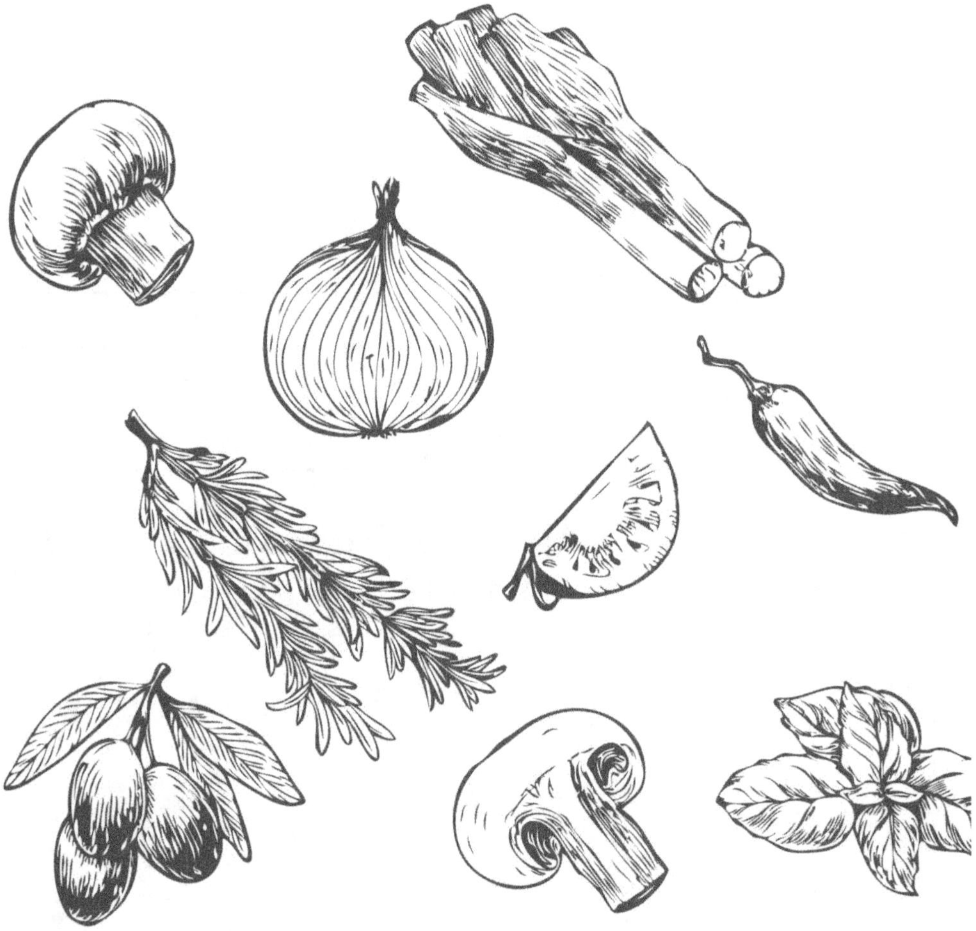

RADISHES & GREEN BEANS

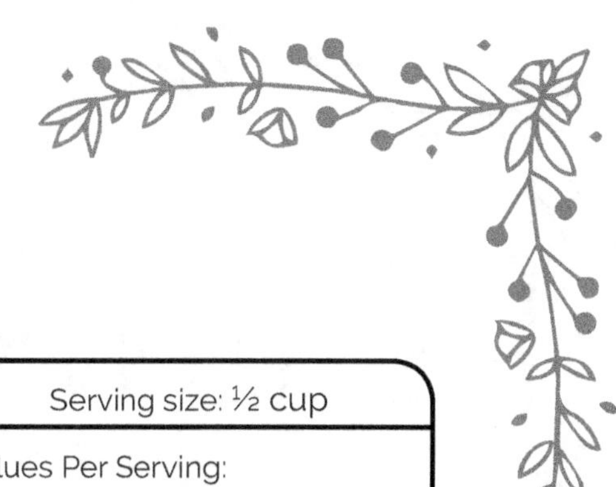

Servings: 4	Serving size: ½ cup

Nutritional Values Per Serving:

Net Carbs:	3 g	Protein:	2 g
Fat:	6 g	Calories:	75 kcal

Ingredients

1 tbsp butter

2 cups green beans

1 cup radishes, thinly sliced

½ tsp sweetener

2 tbsp pine nuts

This is how you make the recipe

1. Heat the butter in a pan, add the beans, stir while cooking for 4 minutes.

2. Add the radishes and continue stirring while cooking for 3 more minutes.

3. Add the sweetener and salt to taste.

4. Sprinkle with pine nuts.

GARBANZO STUFFED PEPPERS

Yield: 32

Nutritional Values Per Serving:

Net Carbs:	2 g	Protein:	1 g
Fat:	0 g	Calories:	15 kcal

Ingredients

16 small sweet peppers, sliced in half

1 tsp cumin seeds

2½ cups garbanzo beans, rinsed and drained

¼ cup coriander leaves

3 tbsp apple cider vinegar

This is how you make the recipe

1. Toast cumin seeds in a pan over medium heat for about 1-2 minutes, stir occasionally.

2. Pour the garbanzo beans, cilantro, vinegar and the cumin seeds in a blender; add 3 tbsp of water and add salt to taste. Pulse until smooth.

3. Spoon into pepper halves and enjoy!

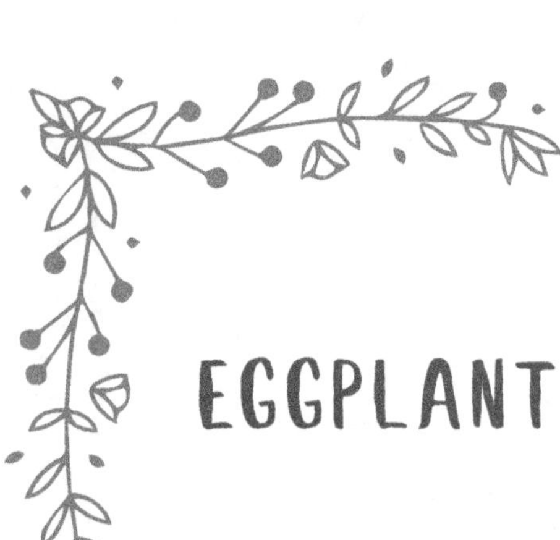

EGGPLANT SAVORY

Ingredients

2 cups eggplant

2 tbsp butter

4 eggs

3 cups almond milk

¼ cup dried cranberries

This is how you make the recipe

1. Preheat the oven to 350˚F.

2. Cut the eggplant into ¾-inch slices. Spread them out onto paper towels, sprinkle salt over them and let sit for 8 minutes. Dry off the water on top of the eggplant.

3. Line a baking dish with parchment paper and place eggplant in it.

4. Drizzle melted butter over the eggplant.

5. Bake for 15 minutes, then drain off any extra liquid.

6. Blend together the eggs, almond milk and a little salt until well-combined.

7. Pour the milk mixture over eggplant.

8. Sprinkle cranberries on top.

9. Bake for 45 minutes.

10. Serve warm and enjoy.

NUT PUDDING

Ingredients

1 cup heavy cream

1 cup mascarpone cheese, softened

1 cup cottage cheese

¼ cup chopped walnuts

1 tsp beef gelatin

This is how you make the recipe

1. Beat the double cream until stiff.

2. Fold in the mascarpone.

3. Stir in the cottage cheese and gelatin and mix well.

4. Fold in the walnuts.

5. Spoon into small bowls and let chill for four hours before serving.

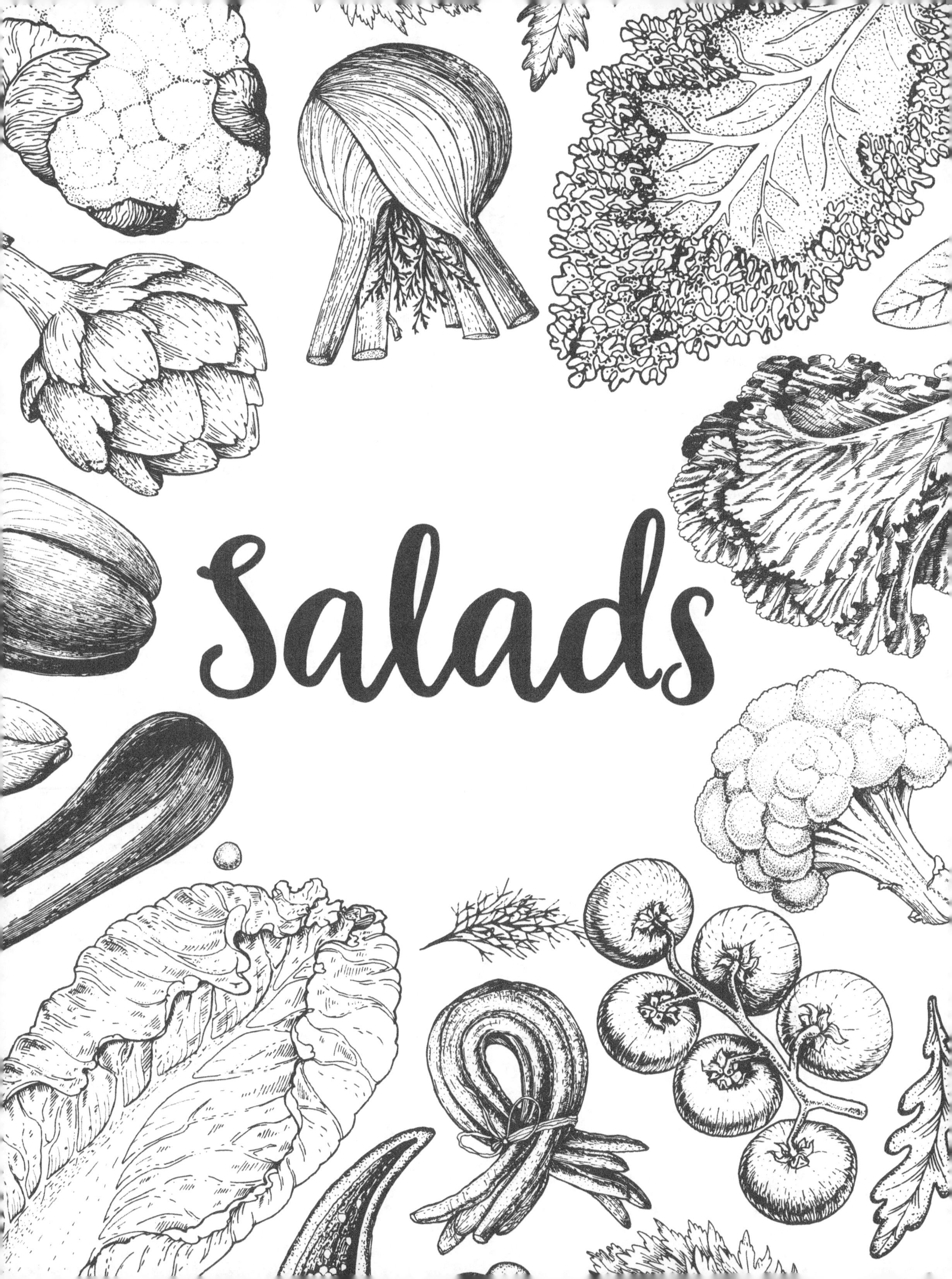
Salads

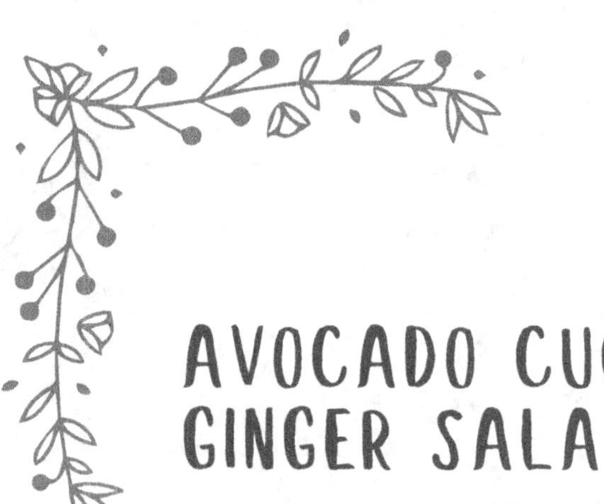

AVOCADO CUCUMBER GINGER SALAD

Ingredients

½ cucumber, peeled and diced small

½ avocado, diced small

1 tbsp ginger, grated

1 tsp lemon juice

1 tbsp olive oil

This is how you make the recipe

1. Mix the diced cucumber, avocado, and grated ginger.

2. Toss with olive oil and salt to taste.

3. Tip: You can top it with goji berries for a nice taste and decoration.

BLUEBERRY CHICKEN SALAD

Ingredients

10 blueberries

¼ onion, sliced

5 cups lettuce leaves

2 tsp lemon juice

1 boneless, skinless chicken breast half

This is how you make the recipe

1. Sauté the diced chicken breast in 2 tbsp of oil. Add salt and pepper to taste.

2. In a salad bowl, toss the cooked chicken with the blueberries, onion slices, salad leaves, olive oil, and lemon juice. Enjoy!

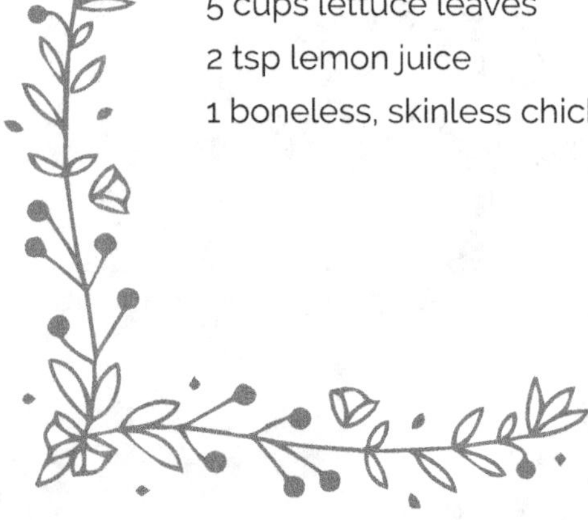

TOMATO MOZZARELLA SALAD

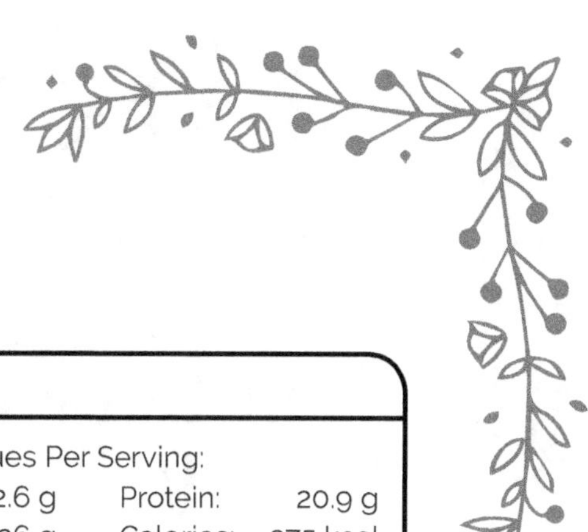

Servings: 10

Nutritional Values Per Serving:

Net Carbs:	12.6 g	Protein:	20.9 g
Fat:	26 g	Calories:	375 kcal

Ingredients

5 tomatoes

2 balls of mozzarella cheese, sliced

10 basil leaves, roughly cut

½ cup balsamic vinegar

Olive oil

This is how you make the recipe

1. Slice the tomatoes and spread them out on a plate.

2. Lay the cheese slices and the basil leaves onto the tomatoes.

3. Drizzle on the oil and vinegar then sprinkle on salt to taste.

GARDEN ROCKET STRAWBERRY SALAD

Servings: 2

Nutritional Values Per Serving:

Net Carbs:	5 g	Protein:	4 g
Fat:	21 g	Calories:	228 kcal

Ingredients

4 cups baby arugula

6 strawberries, quartered

¼ cup almonds, toasted & sliced

2 tbsp lemon juice

This is how you make the recipe

1. Layer arugula, strawberries, almonds on a plate.

2. Drizzle with lemon juice and oil and vinegar.

3. Add salt and pepper to taste.

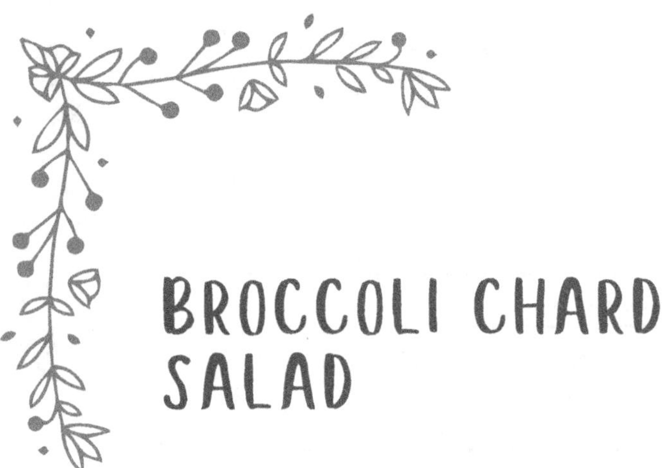

BROCCOLI CHARD SALAD

Servings: 4

Nutritional Values Per Serving:
Net Carbs: 15 g   Protein: 8 g
Fat: 11,6 g   Calories: 221 kcal

Ingredients

8 cups chard leaves, chopped

4 cups broccoli

20 cherry tomatoes

4 cucumbers

2 avocados

This is how you make the recipe

1. Steam the broccoli for 5 minutes.

2. Slice and cut the cucumbers into half circle slices.

3. Cut the cherry tomatoes in half.

4. Slice the avocados.

5. Mix all together in a salad bowl and top with dressing of your choice. Enjoy!

AVOCADO TUNA SALAD

Servings: 6

Nutritional Values Per Serving:
Net Carbs: 4 g   Protein: 22 g
Fat: 20 g   Calories: 304 kcal

Ingredients

3 small cans tuna, drained

1 cucumber, sliced

2 avocados, sliced

1 red onion, thinly sliced

¼ cup cilantro

This is how you make the recipe

1. In a large salad bowl, combine the cucumber, avocado, onion, tuna, and cilantro .

2. Drizzle with oil and vinegar, salt and pepper to taste.

3. Toss to combine and serve.

CREAMY DILL CUCUMBER SALAD

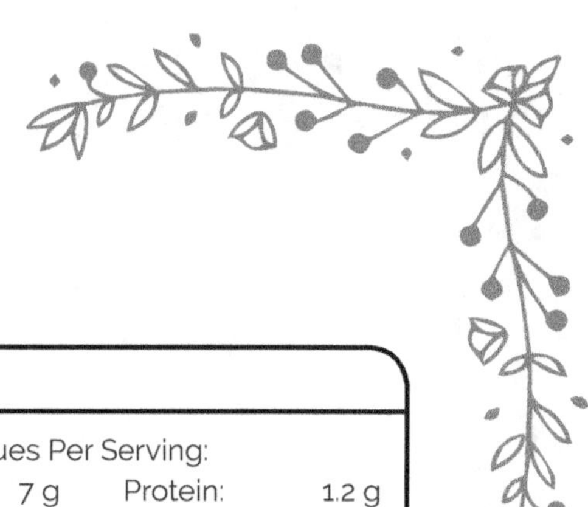

Servings: 4

Nutritional Values Per Serving:

| Net Carbs: | 7 g | Protein: | 1.2 g |
| Fat: | 1 g | Calories: | 47 kcal |

Ingredients

2 large cucumbers, sliced

¼ cup red onion, sliced

¼ cup Greek yogurt (or sour cream or mayo or combination)

1 lemon, juice and zest

2 tbsp dill, chopped

This is how you make the recipe

1. Mix everything together in a salad bowl.

2. Add salt and pepper to taste

3. Enjoy!

FETA LEMON COLESLAW

Servings: 4

Nutritional Values Per Serving:

| Net Carbs: | 5 g | Protein: | 4 g |
| Fat: | 14 g | Calories: | 165 kcal |

Ingredients

½ head white cabbage, finely sliced

Juice from ½ lemon

3 tbsp olive oil

½ cup feta cheese, crumbled

2 spring onions, finely chopped

This is how you make the recipe

1. Place the white cabbage and green onion in a bowl.

2. Blend the feta cheese, lemon and olive oil in a bowl. Add the salt and pepper to taste.

3. Pour over the cabbage and toss until covered.

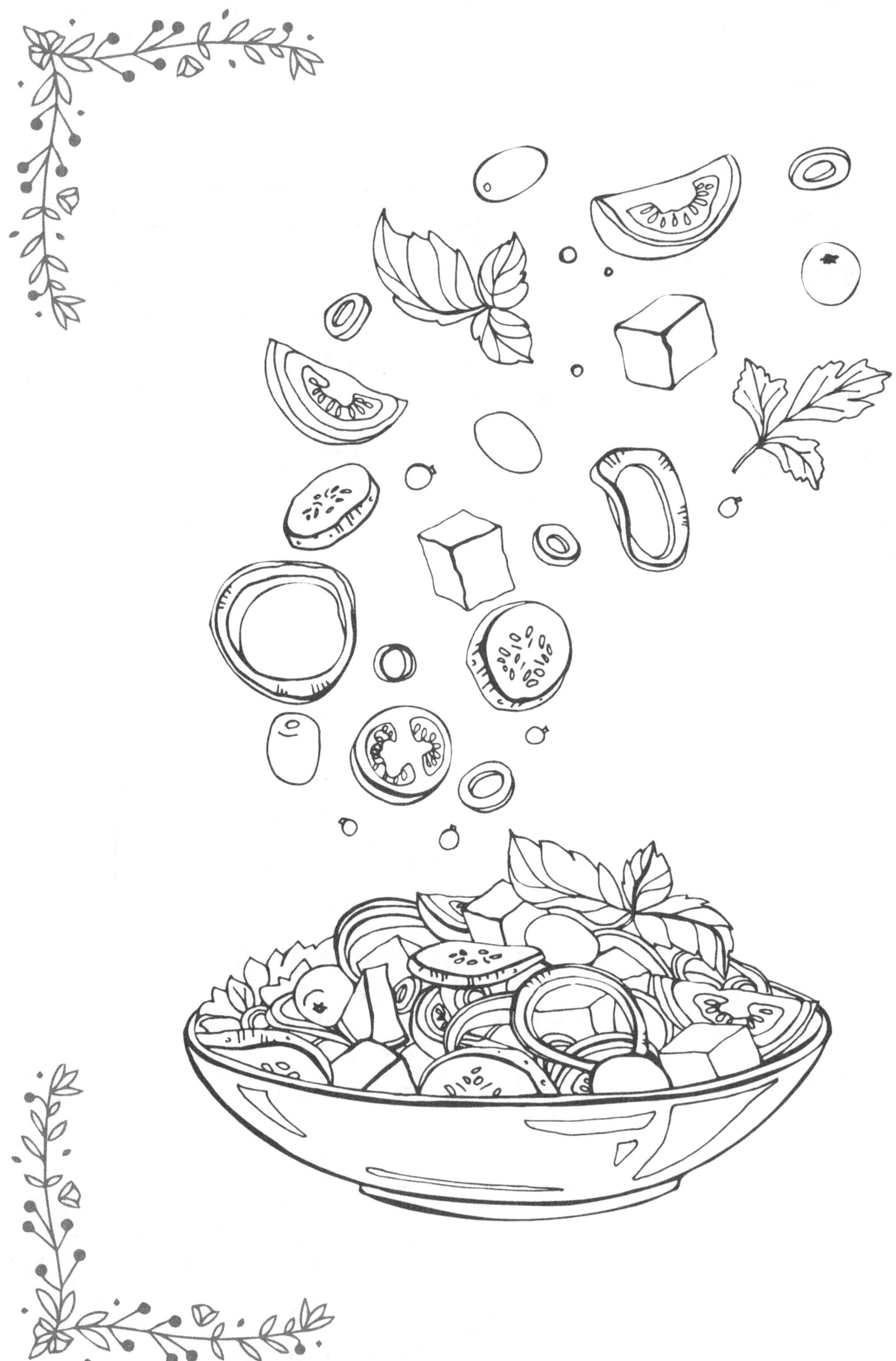

CHICKEN SALAD

<table>
<tr><td>Servings: 2</td></tr>
</table>

Nutritional Values Per Serving:

Net Carbs:	3.14 g	Protein:	38.7 g
Fat:	43.8 g	Calories:	581 kcal

Ingredients

2 boneless chicken breasts halves, with skin

6 slices of bacon

1 avocado, sliced

4 cups mixed leafy greens

4 tbsp ranch dressing or dressing of choice

This is how you make the recipe

1. Preheat the oven to 400˚F.

2. Season the chicken breasts with salt and pepper.

3. In an oiled, hot frying pan, place the chicken breasts, skin side down.

4. Cook the chicken for 6 minutes until golden brown and crispy. Then flip the chicken on the other side and continue cooking for another minute. Then place the pan in the oven.

5. Bake the chicken for 15 minutes or until the internal temperature reaches at least 73˚C.

6. Cook the bacon until crispy.

7. Remove the chicken to a cutting board and let sit for 5 minutes.

8. Slice the chicken and the avocado.

9. Place the greens in a bowl, then add avocado, bacon and chicken.

10. Top with the dressing and enjoy!

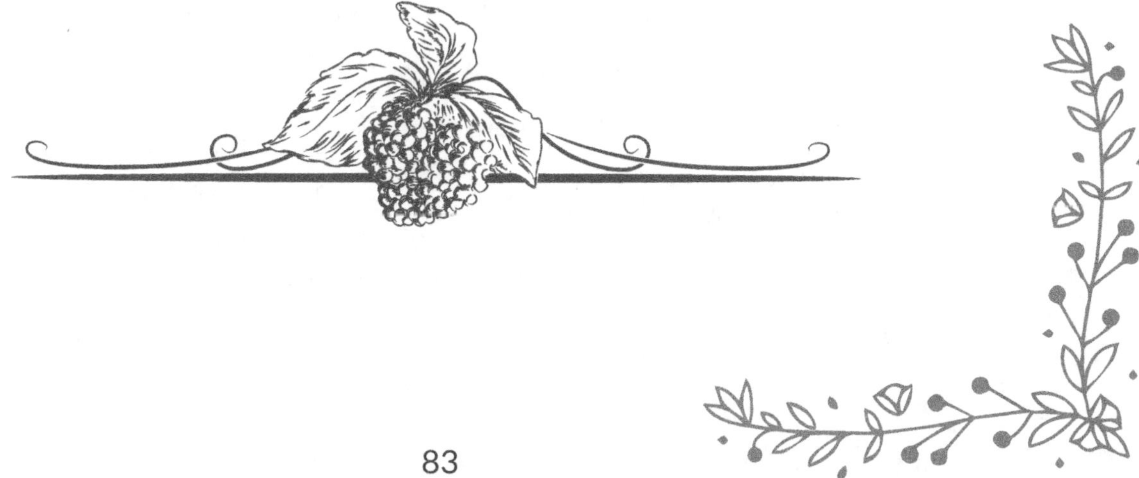

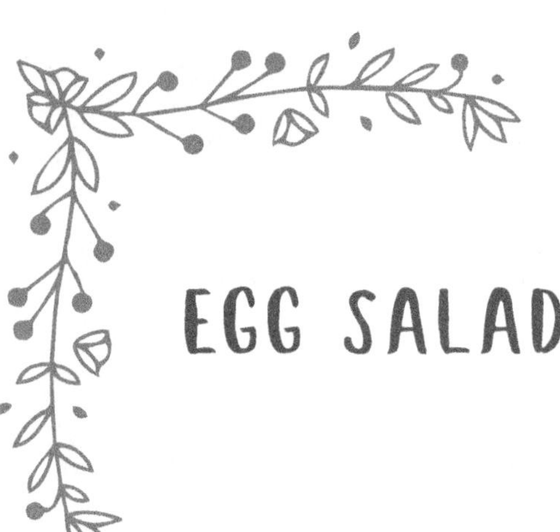

EGG SALAD

Yield: 1 ½ cups   Serving size: ¼ cup

Nutritional Values Per Serving:
Net Carbs: 1 g   Protein: 7 g
Fat: 22 g   Calories: 217 kcal

Ingredients

7 eggs, hard boiled, finely chopped
½ cup mayonnaise
1 tsp mustard
¼ cup spring onions, thinly sliced
2 stalks of celery, finely chopped

This is how you make the recipe

1. Add all ingredients to a medium sized bowl until thoroughly combined.

2. Adjust seasoning as desired.

3. Refrigerate or serve immediately.

4. Garnish with extra spring onions.

GRILLED EGGPLANT SALAD

Servings: 4

Nutritional Values Per Serving:
Net Carbs: 9 g   Protein: 15 g
Fat: 47 g   Calories: 532 kcal

Ingredients

2 eggplants
½ cup olive oil
2 tbsp lemon juice
1 can of tuna
1 ball of mozzarella cheese, sliced

This is how you make the recipe

1. Slice the eggplant and sprinkle with salt. Place the slices on paper towels for 8 minutes.

2. Cook both sides of the eggplant slices in an oiled pan until very soft.

3. Mix the olive oil and lemon juice. Add minced garlic (optional).

4. Pour the dressing on a plate and lay the eggplant slices in it to soak.

5. Spread the tuna over the slices.

6. Lay slices of the mozzarella on top.

7. Sprinkle with olive oil and lemon juice, season with pepper.

KALE AND BLUEBERRY SALAD

Servings: 4

Nutritional Values Per Serving:

Net Carbs:	13 g	Protein:	4 g
Fat:	16 g	Calories:	191 kcal

Ingredients

12 oz kale

20 blueberries

2 tbsp almonds, sliced

½ onion, thinly sliced

2 tbsp lemon juice

This is how you make the recipe

1. Roughly chop the kale. Throw it into a salad bowl.

2. Drop in the almonds and onion and blueberries.

3. Drizzle on the lemon juice and salt and pepper to taste.

4. Toss and enjoy.

TUNA SALAD

Servings: 2

Nutritional Values Per Serving:

Net Carbs:	3 g	Protein:	45 g
Fat:	40 g	Calories:	480 kcal

Ingredients

1 cucumber

1 avocado

2 tsp lemon juice

1 can of tuna

2 tbsp mayo

This is how you make the recipe

1. Dice cucumber and avocado.

2. Mix the cucumber and avocado with the lemon juice.

3. Combine the tuna with the mayonnaise.

4. Add the tuna mixture to the avocado and cucumber.

5. Salt and pepper to taste.

SHRIMP & CAULIFLOWER

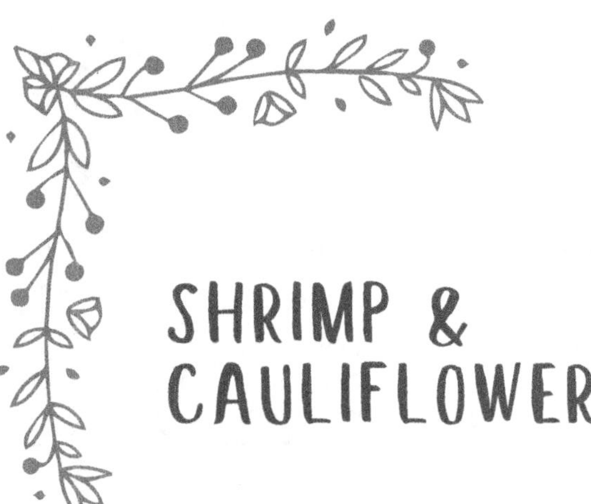

Ingredients

1 head of cauliflower, cut into small florets

3 cups shrimp, peeled and deveined

2 cucumbers, thinly sliced

3 tbsp dill, chopped

⅓ cup olive oil

This is how you make the recipe

1. Put the shrimp in an oiled pan. Salt and pepper to taste and cook until opaque.

2. Steam the cauliflower florets for 15 minutes, until tender.

3. Slice the shrimps in half.

4. Combine the shrimp, cauliflower, and cucumber slices in a bowl.

5. Pour the olive oil over it, sprinkle on the dill and add salt and pepper to taste.

6. Toss and serve.

ROCKET SHRIMP SALAD

Ingredients

8 cups baby arugula, roughly chopped

3 cups large shrimp, peeled, deveined and cooked

1 avocado, diced

4 tbsp olive oil

2 lemons, 1 juiced and 1 cut into wedges

This is how you make the recipe

1. Place the arugula, shrimp, and avocado in a bowl.

2. Sprinkle with half of the olive oil, lemon juice and salt and pepper to taste.

3. Toss and serve with the lemon wedges.

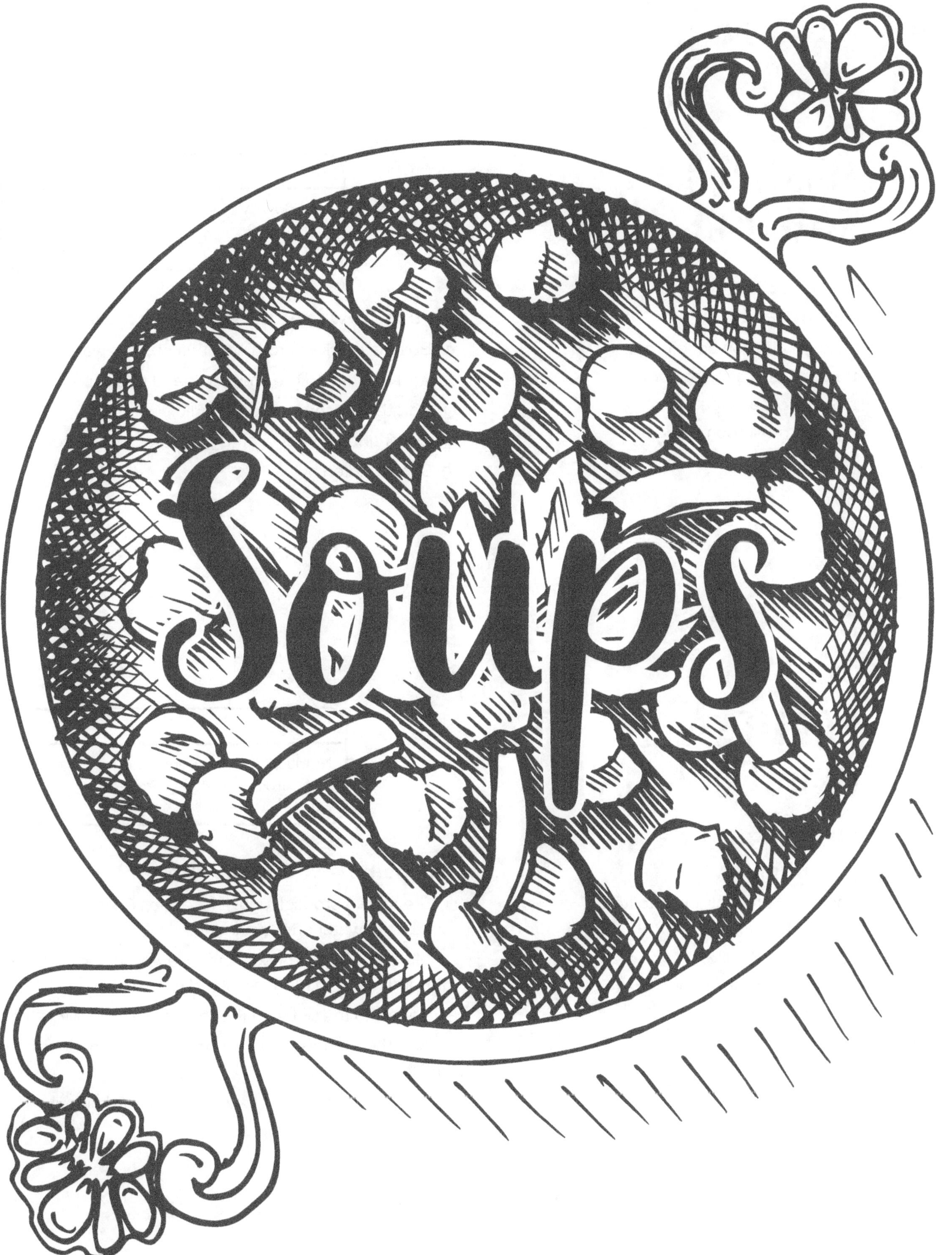
Soups

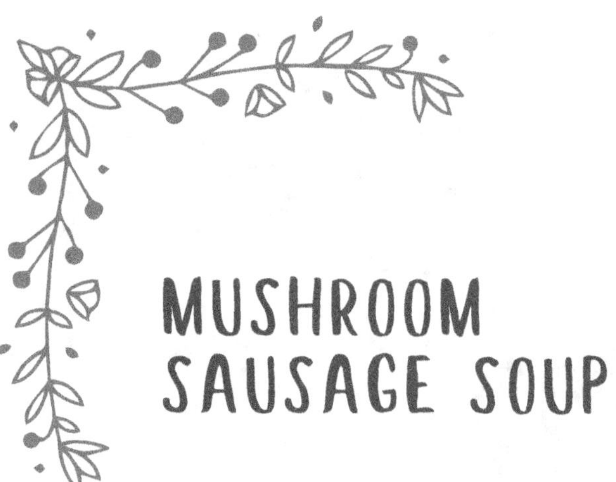

MUSHROOM SAUSAGE SOUP

Ingredients

3½ cups chicken bone broth

1½ cups kale, chopped small

12 slices of sausage

1¼ cups mushrooms, slices

2 cloves garlic

This is how you make the recipe

1. Boil the chicken broth with two cups of water.
2. Add the kale to the soup. Salt and pepper to taste.
3. Add the mushrooms and garlic.
4. Cover and simmer over low heat for half an hour.
5. Serve and enjoy!

PARMESAN BROCCOLI SOUP

Ingredients

2 heads of broccoli, cut into florets

2 cups of water

1 cup almond milk

½ cup parmesan cheese, grated

1 tbsp lemon juice

This is how you make the recipe

1. Steam the broccoli until it is tender. Reserve one cup of the water after steaming.
2. Mix half of the broccoli, the reserved water and the almond milk in a blender. Blend until smooth.
3. Return to the pot with the rest of the broccoli.
4. Add the parmesan and lemon juice and heat up until hot.
5. Add salt and pepper to taste, serve and enjoy!

TOMATO BASIL SOUP

Servings: 6

Nutritional Values Per Serving:

| Net Carbs: | 2 g | Protein: | 28 g |
| Fat: | 3 g | Calories: | 287 kcal |

Ingredients

5 cups tomato puree

1 stick of salted butter

1 cup cream cheese

Handful of basil leaves

1 tbsp sweetener

This is how you make the recipe

1. Pour the puree into a large saucepan. Add the butter and cream cheese.

2. Heat to a simmer and cook until the butter and cream cheese melt.

3. Carefully pour the soup into a blender, add the basil and sweetener to blend.

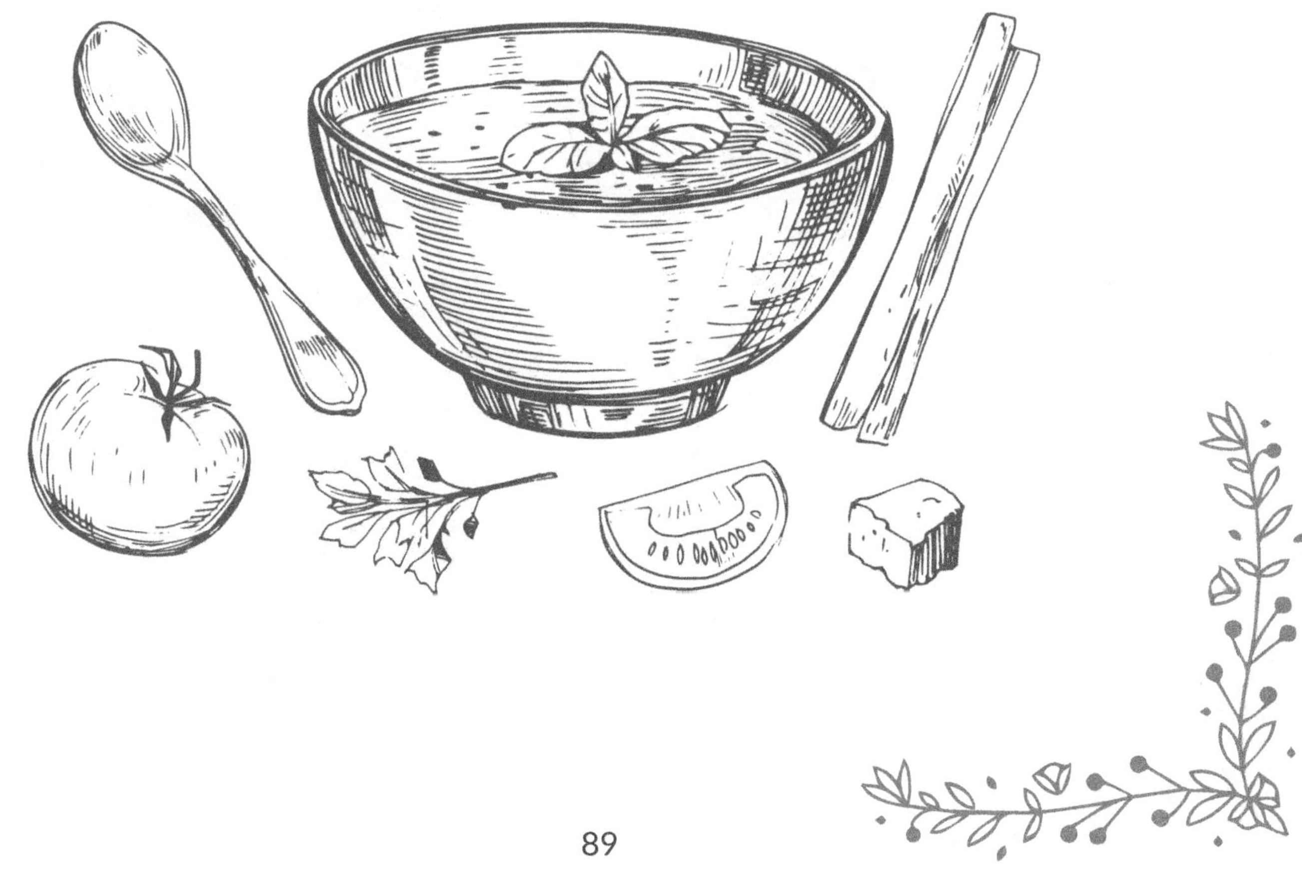

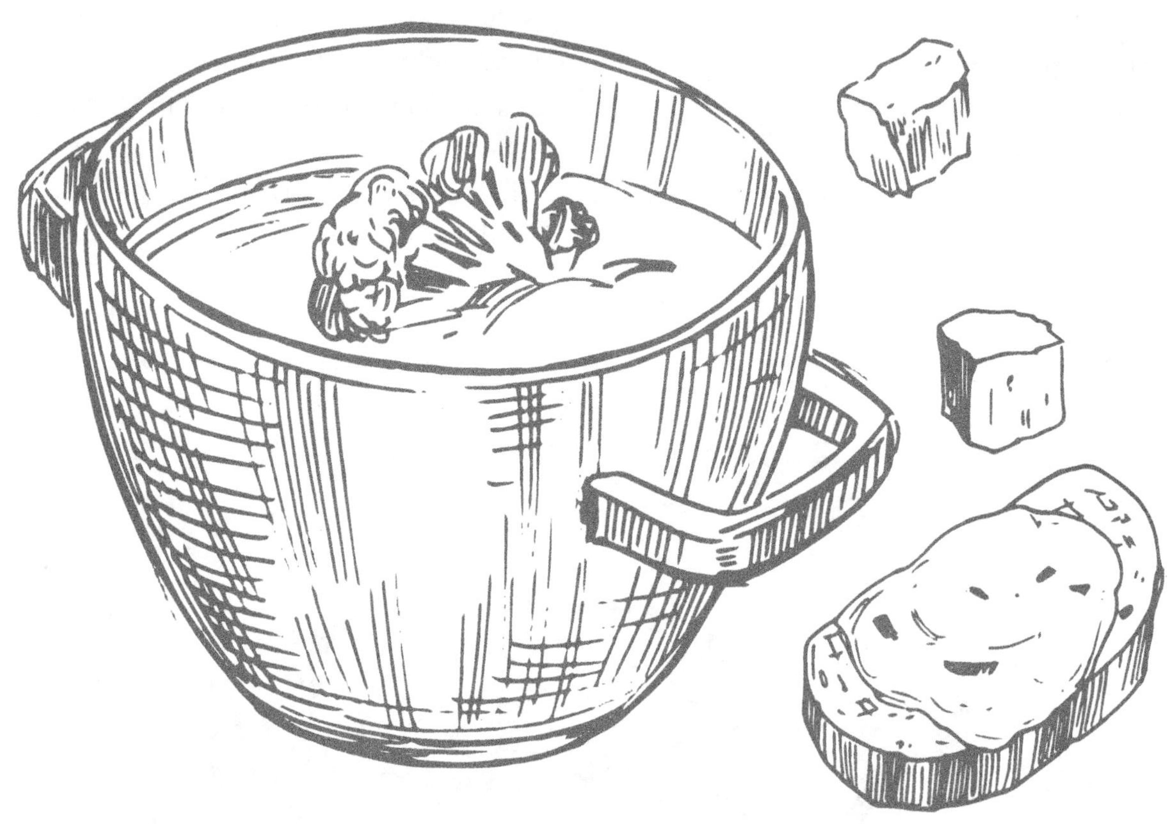

BROCCOLI SOUP

Ingredients

4 cups broccoli florets
2 cloves garlic
4 cups chicken broth
1 cup heavy cream
2 cups mozzarella

This is how you make the recipe

1. Cook the garlic in a pot, add the broth, chopped broccoli and heavy cream.

2. On low heat, let simmer for 15 minutes, until broccoli is soft.

3. Add minced garlic, turmeric, salt, pepper. Gradually add the mozzarella.

4. Keep stirring until melted.

5. Remove from the oven.

6. Mix it to make it creamy and serve.

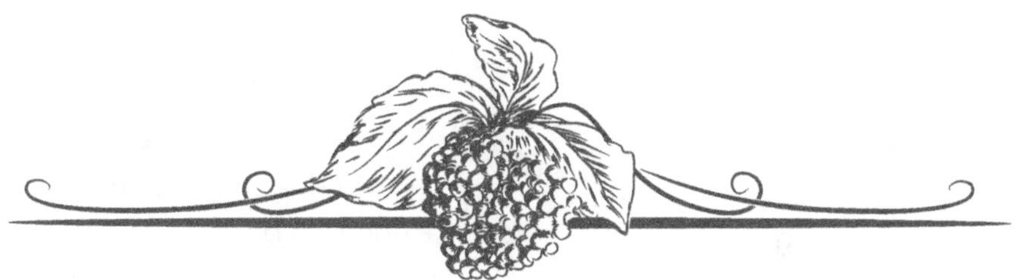

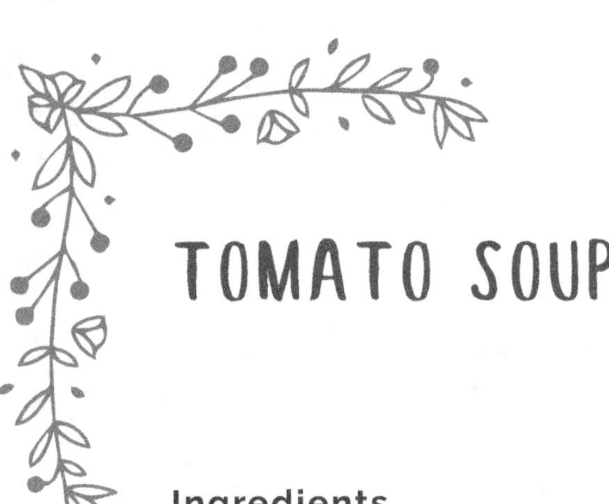

TOMATO SOUP

Ingredients

1 tin whole plum tomatoes
¼ tsp garlic, minced
1 cup mascarpone cheese
1 tsp apple cider vinegar
¼ cup basil pesto

This is how you make the recipe

1. In a pot, combine the tomatoes, one cup of water, garlic and add salt to taste.

2. Bring to a boil and then let simmer for 5 minutes.

3. Remove from the oven and puree until smooth.

4. Return to the stove and add mascarpone cheese in small pieces to the soup.

5. Stir for 2 minutes, until melted.

6. Stir in the apple cider vinegar, the pesto and add sweetener to taste.

CHICKEN FEET BONE BROTH

Ingredients

12 chicken feet
2 tbsp apple cider vinegar
1 sprig rosemary
1 piece ginger, ½-inch long
1 clove garlic

This is how you make the recipe

1. Add chicken feet and apple cider vinegar with water in a pot.

2. Bring water to boil, then let simmer for 10 minutes.

3. Strain and rinse off the feet in cold water, pull off any leftover membranes.

4. Add the chicken feet to a pot and add filtered water. Bring to a boil.

5. Reduce the heat and let simmer. Skim off any scum.

6. Add the ginger, rosemary, garlic and add salt to taste.

7. Let simmer for 8-10 hours.

8. Strain the liquid into glass jars and serve immediately.

Fat Bombs

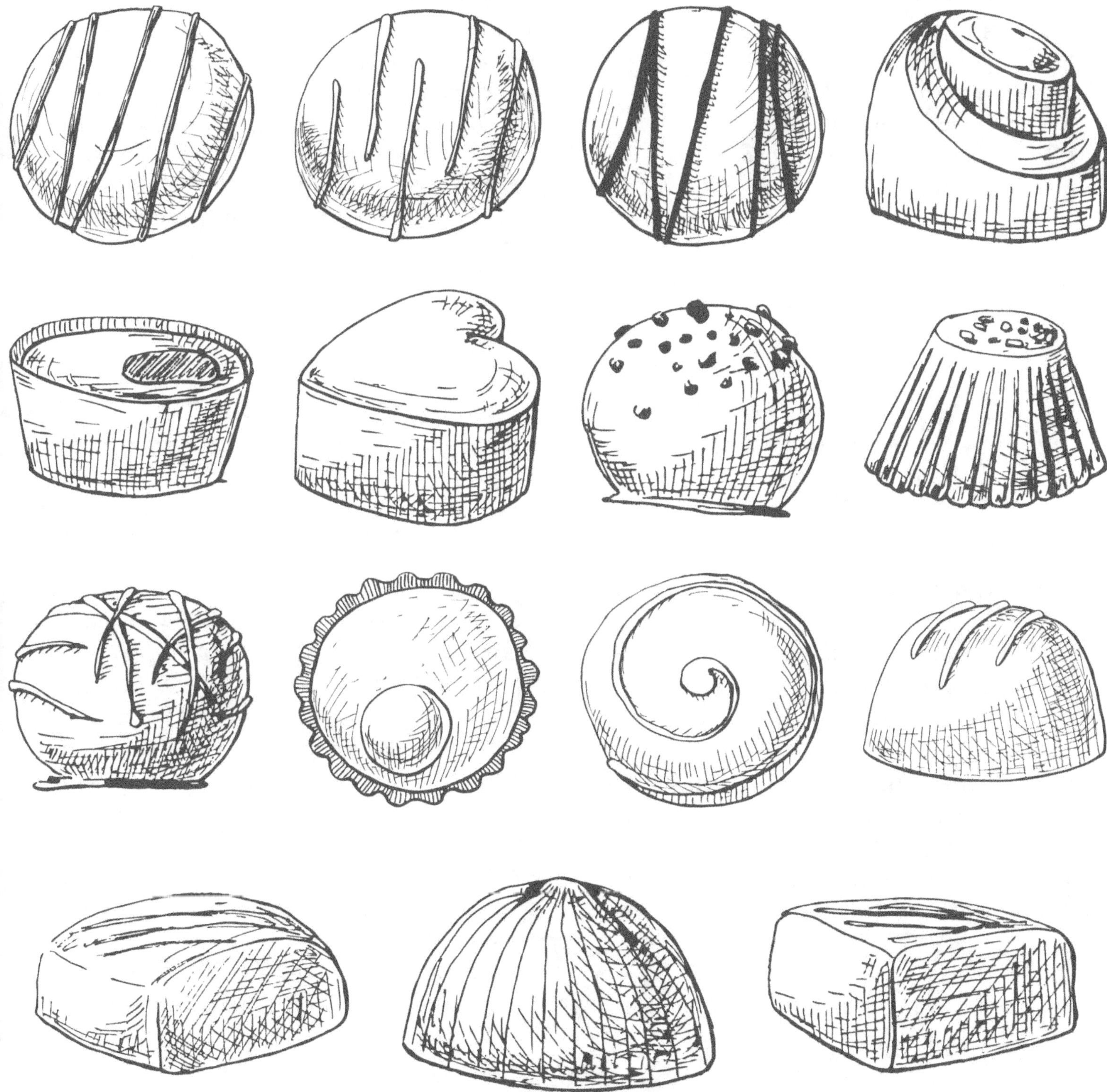

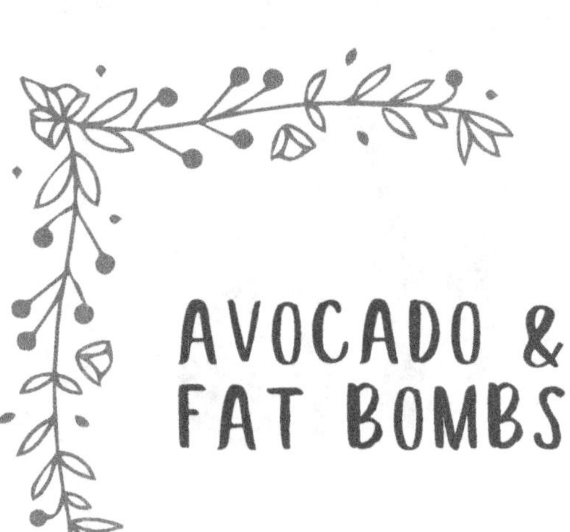

AVOCADO & EGG FAT BOMBS

Servings: 5

Nutritional Values Per Serving:
Net Carbs: 1.1 g   Protein: 2.2 g
Fat: 14.8 g   Calories: 147 kcal

Ingredients

3 eggs
½ avocado
¼ cup mayonnaise
1 tbsp lemon or lime juice
2 tbsp spring onions, chopped

This is how you make the recipe

1. Hard boil the eggs.

2. Peel and carefully cut the eggs in half. Spoon the egg yolks into a bowl.

3. Place the avocado into a food processor and add the egg yolks, mayonnaise, lemon juice. Salt and pepper to taste. Process until smooth.

4. Spoon the mixture back into the egg white halves and serve.

5. Enjoy with spring onion on top.

BACON & EGG FAT BOMBS

Servings: 6

Nutritional Values Per Serving:
Net Carbs: 0.2 g   Protein: 5 g
Fat: 18.4 g   Calories: 185 kcal

Ingredients

2 eggs
¼ cup butter, softened
2 tbsp mayonnaise
4 slices of bacon

This is how you make the recipe

1. Preheat the oven to 375 ˚F. Line a baking tray with greaseproof paper.

2. Lay the slices of bacon on the greaseproof paper, leaving space so they don't overlap.

3. Place the sheet in the oven and cook for about 10-15 minutes until golden brown. Remove from the oven and set aside to cool down.

4. Hard boil the eggs. Cut into quarters.

5. Cut the butter into small pieces and add the eggs. Mash with a fork.

6. Add the mayonnaise, salt and pepper to taste and mix well.

7. Pour in the bacon grease and combine well.

8. Place in the fridge for half an hour until they harden enough to form balls.

9. Crumble the bacon and place it on a plate.

10. Roll each ball in the bacon crumbles and place on a tray to enjoy.

FUDGY MACADAMIA FAT BOMB

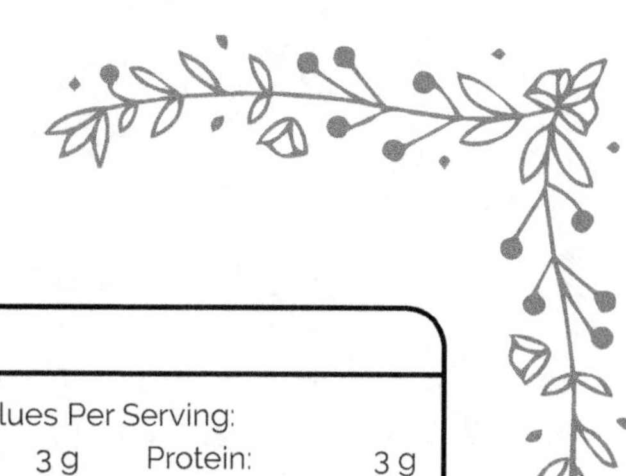

Servings: 6

Nutritional Values Per Serving:

Net Carbs:	3 g	Protein:	3 g
Fat:	28 g	Calories:	267 kcal

Ingredients

¼ cup cocoa butter

2 tbsp cocoa powder

2 tbsp sweetener

¼ cup macadamia nuts, chopped

¼ cup heavy cream

This is how you make the recipe

1. Melt the cocoa butter in a double boiler.

2. Add the cocoa powder and the sweetener. Mix well until all is well blended.

3. Add the macadamia nuts and stir in well.

4. Add the cream, mix and then bring up the temperature to ensure all remains are well melted.

5. Pour into a mold.

6. Let cool then put in the fridge to harden.

BROWNIE BALLS

Servings: 30

Nutritional Values Per Serving:

Net Carbs:	1.4 g	Protein:	1.9 g
Fat:	4.4 g	Calories:	51 kcal

Ingredients

1 cup nut butter of choice

⅔ cup unsweetened cocoa powder

5 tbsp sweetener

½ cup chocolate chips

2 tbsp coconut oil

This is how you make the recipe

1. Except for the chocolate chips, blend everything together in a food processor, until it forms a smooth dough. You may want to add a pinch of salt to taste.

2. Place in the fridge until the dough firms up.

3. Spoon portions out and roll into balls.

4. Press in a couple of chocolate chips into each ball and enjoy.

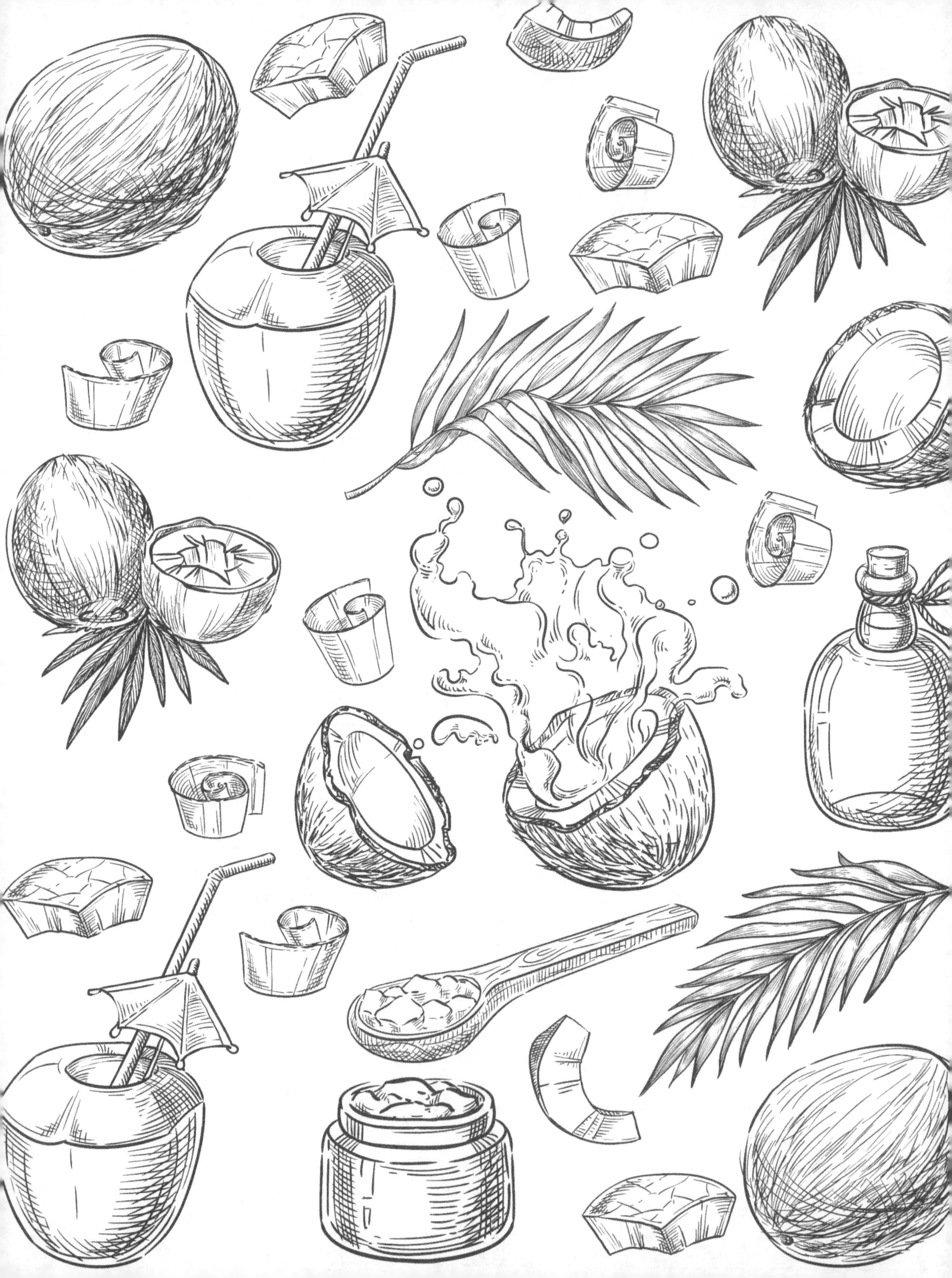

COCONUT FAT BOMBS

Servings: 12

Nutritional Values Per Serving:
Net Carbs: 0.74 g Protein: 1.9 g
Fat: 9.6 g Calories: 104 kcal

Ingredients

1½ cup coconut flakes
¼ cup coconut oil
¼ tsp vanilla extract
¼ cup confectioners' sweetener
Pinch of salt

This is how you make the recipe

1. Preheat the oven to 350 ˚F.

2. Spread the coconut on a baking sheet. Place in the oven and toast for 5 minutes, until light golden. Stir as needed to prevent burning.

3. Transfer into a blender and pulse until smooth.

4. Add the butter and coconut oil.

5. Add the vanilla, sweetener and salt and mix well.

6. Pour into a mold.

7. Place in the fridge for at least 30 minutes and let it solidify.

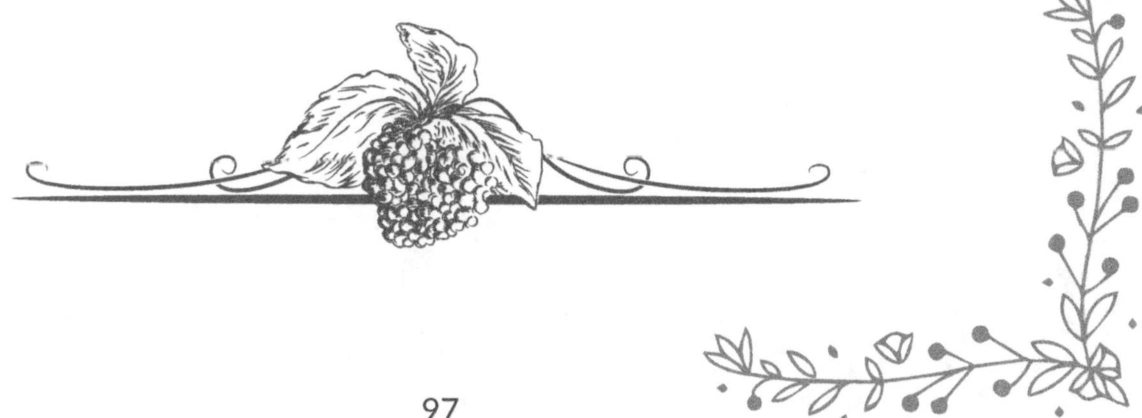

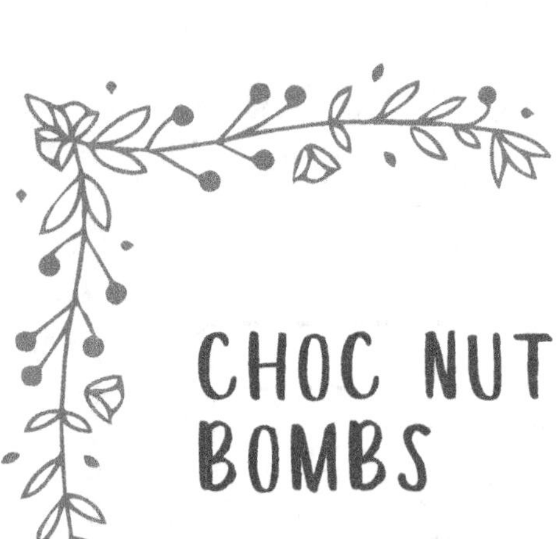

CHOC NUT FAT BOMBS

Ingredients

1 cup melted coconut oil

1 cup cocoa powder

1 cup almond butter

This is how you make the recipe

1. Melt the coconut oil and whisk in the cocoa and almond butter until no lumps remain.

2. Spoon 1 tbsp of the mixture each into molds.

3. Refrigerate or freeze until hard.

4. Enjoy! Store in the refrigerator.

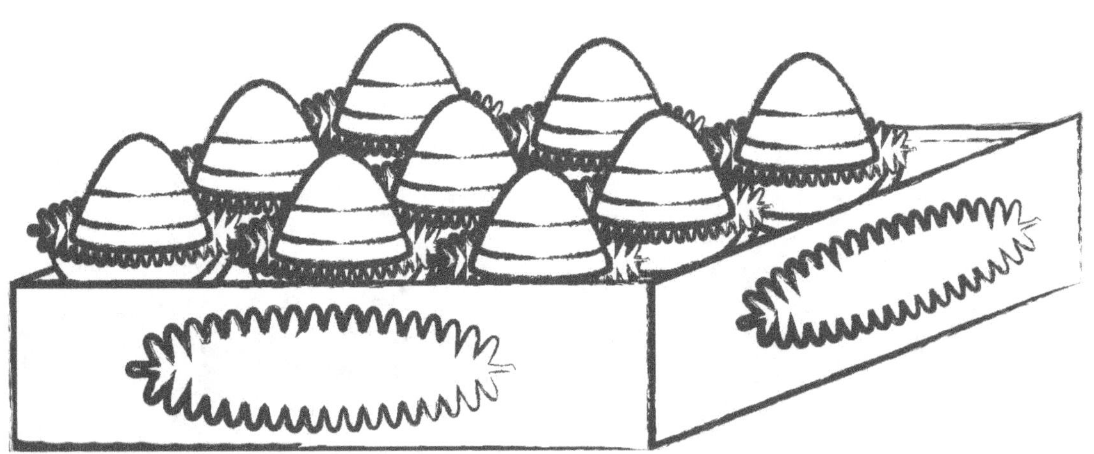

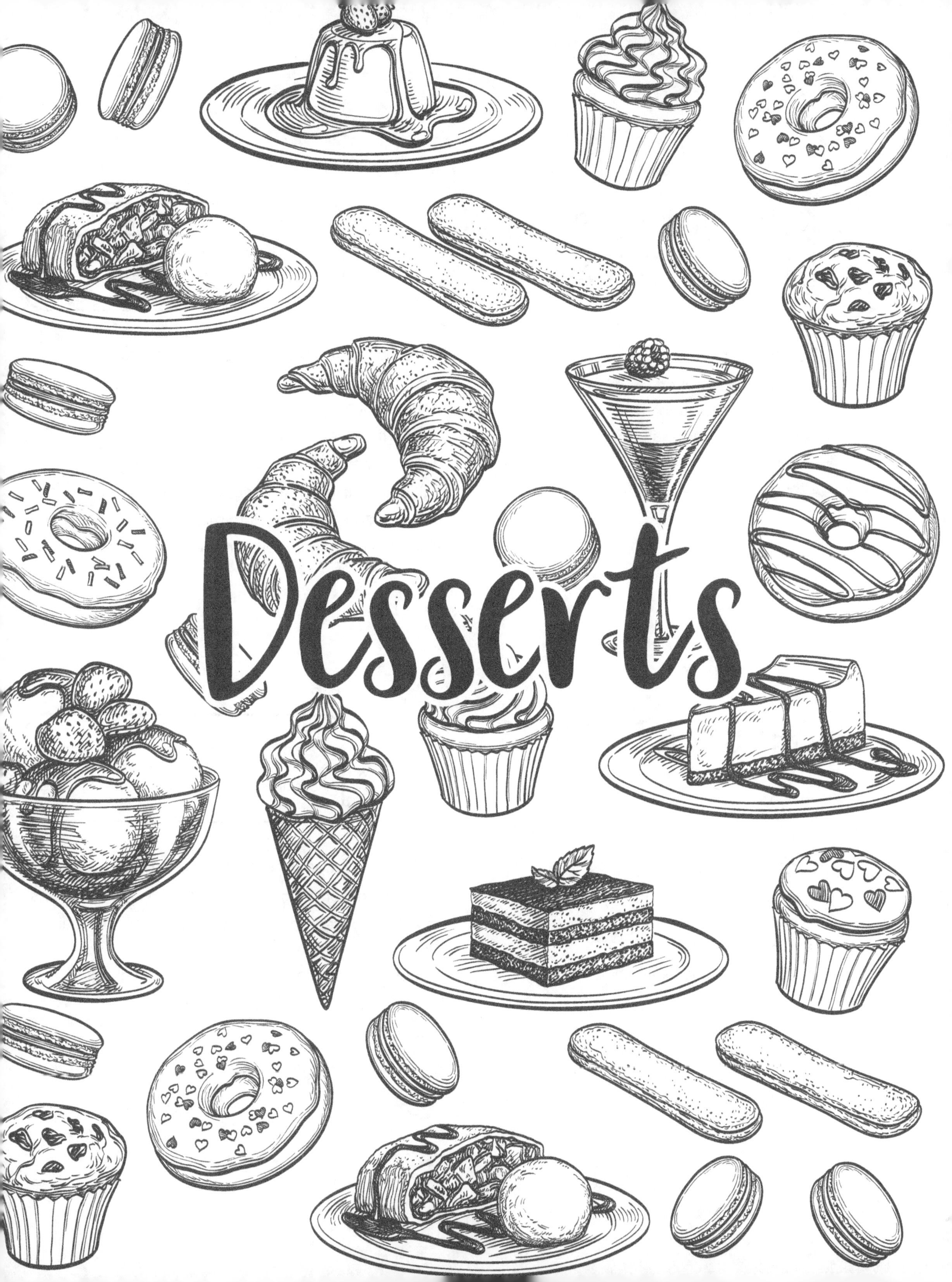

Desserts

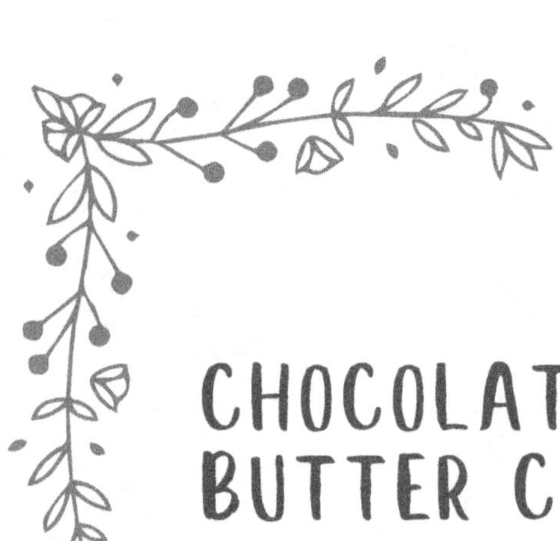

CHOCOLATE ALMOND BUTTER CUPS

Yield: 6 cups

Nutritional Values Per Serving:

Net Carbs:	1.5 g	Protein:	3 g
Fat:	26 g	Calories:	263 kcal

Ingredients

4 tbsp almond butter

1 stick unsalted butter

⅓ cup baking chocolate

⅓ cup sweetener

2 tbsp heavy cream

This is how you make the recipe

1. Melt the chocolate with the unsalted butter in a double boiler.

2. Add the sweetener.

3. Stir in the cream and the almond butter.

4. Line a muffin pan with cupcake papers.

5. Portion out the chocolate mixture into the pan.

6. Freeze for 30 minutes or more, until firm and enjoy!

CHOCOLATE MOUSSE

Yield: 4

Nutritional Values Per Serving:

Net Carbs:	7 g	Protein:	5 g
Fat:	35 g	Calories:	372 kcal

Ingredients

1½ cup heavy cream

⅓ cup cocoa powder

2 tbsp sweetener

2 tbsp baking chocolate chips

This is how you make the recipe

1. With a mixer, whip the heavy cream until it thickens.

2. Add the sweetener and cocoa powder. Mix again until stiff peaks form.

3. Spoon into a piping bag and pipe into glasses.

4. Sprinkle on chocolate chips and enjoy!

WHITE CHOCOLATE BARS

Servings: 6

Nutritional Values Per Serving:
Net Carbs: 0.6 g Protein: 0 g
Fat: 13.2 g Calories: 123 kcal

Ingredients

½ cup cocoa butter

3 tbsp sweetener

1 tbsp coconut milk powder

1 tsp sunflower lecithin

½ tsp vanilla extract

This is how you make the recipe

1. Melt together the cocoa butter, sweetener and the coconut milk powder in a double boiler.

2. Remove from the heat and stir in the vanilla.

3. Pour into a mold.

4. Refrigerate until solid.

5. Enjoy! Store in the refrigerator.

ALMOND FUDGE BROWNIES

Servings: 16

Nutritional Values Per Serving:
Net Carbs: 2 g Protein: 5 g
Fat: 11 g Calories: 118 kcal

Ingredients

1 cup almond butter

¾ cup confectioners' sweetener

3 large eggs

10 tbsp unsweetened cocoa powder

½ tsp baking powder

This is how you make the recipe

1. Preheat the oven to 325°F.

2. In a food processor, blend the almond butter and sweetener together.

3. Add in the eggs, cocoa powder, baking powder, and a pinch of salt.

4. Transfer the batter to an oiled 9x9-inch baking pan. Smooth with a spatula.

5. Bake for 11 minutes, remove from the oven and allow to cool completely to firm up before cutting.

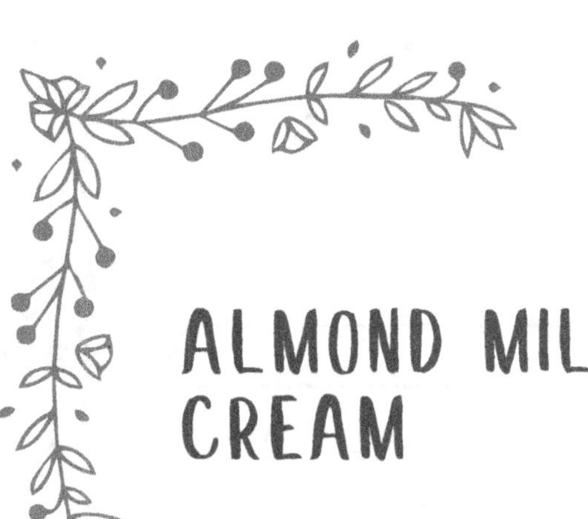

ALMOND MILK ICE CREAM

Ingredients

2 cups almond milk

1 large egg

1 tbsp vanilla extract

½ tbsp gelatin

¾ cup sweetener

This is how you make the recipe

1. Combine the almond milk, whipped egg, vanilla extract, gelatin and sweetener in a saucepan over medium heat. Salt to taste.

2. Let the mixture cook until it begins to steep (strands of steam form on top of the heated liquid).

3. Transfer the liquid to a heat-safe container and place it into your fridge for an hour to cool.

4. Pour it into an ice cream maker and churn it for 30 minutes.

AVOCADO CHOCOLATE MOUSSE

Ingredients

½ cup baking chocolate chips

2 avocados

4 tbsp milk

½ tsp pure vanilla extract

¼ cup sweetener

This is how you make the recipe

1. Melt the chocolate chips in a double boiler.

2. Combine all ingredients in a food processor until completely smooth.

3. Serve and enjoy!

BLACK FOREST CHEESECAKE MOUSSE

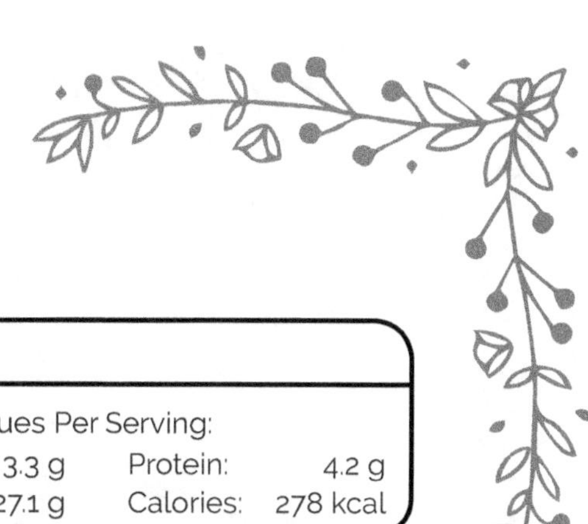

Servings: 6

Nutritional Values Per Serving:
Net Carbs: 3.3 g Protein: 4.2 g
Fat: 27.1 g Calories: 278 kcal

Ingredients

1 cup cream cheese, softened

1 cup heavy cream

¼ cup cocoa powder

½ tsp vanilla extract

¼ cup sweetener

This is how you make the recipe

1. In a blender, mix the cream cheese, cocoa and sweetener until smooth.

2. In a separate bowl, whip the cream until stiff peaks form.

3. Slowly fold the whipped cream into the cream cheese mix.

4. Beat with an electric mixer on high until light and fluffy.

5. Spoon the mixture onto the dessert plates.

6. Refrigerate for at least two hours before serving.

7. Tip: For added flair, top with a cherry.

CHOCOLATE COOKIES

Yield: 12

Nutritional Values Per Serving:
Net Carbs: 2.9 g Protein: 6.8 g
Fat: 14.4 g Calories: 195 kcal

Ingredients

1 ¼ cups almond butter

2 large eggs

⅔ cup cocoa powder

⅓ cup confectioners' sweetener

¼ tsp salt

This is how you make the recipe

1. Preheat the oven to 320°F. Line a baking tray with greaseproof paper.

2. Place the almond butter, eggs, cocoa powder, sweetener and salt into a food processor. Process until well-combined.

3. Create 12 cookie dough balls. Place them on the baking tray.

4. Using a fork, flatten the cookie until they're ½-inch thick.

5. Bake for 12 minutes or until they get crispy.

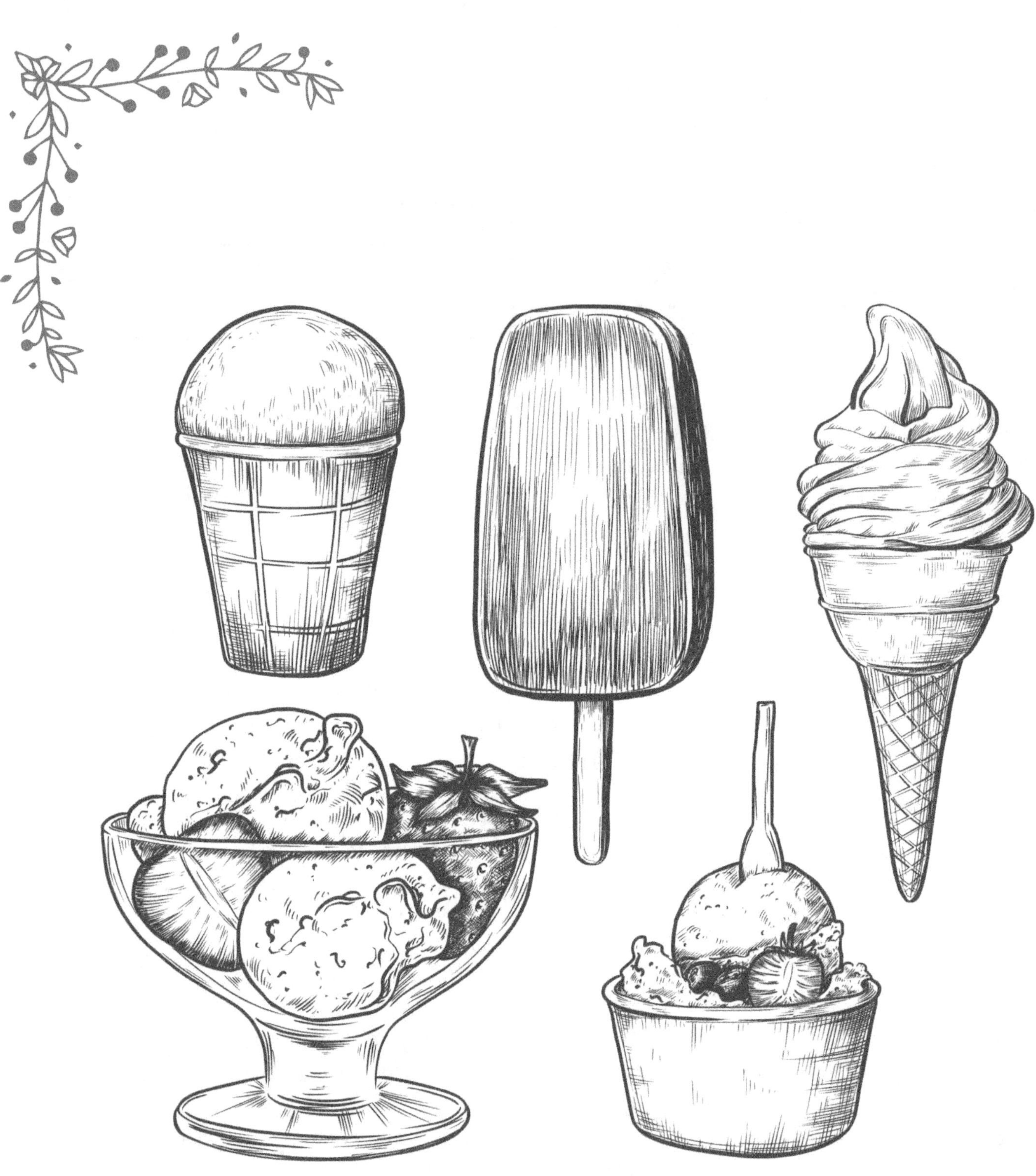

CHOCOLATE ICE CREAM

Servings: 8

Nutritional Values Per Serving:
| Net Carbs: | 7 g | Protein: | 1 g |
| Fat: | 11 g | Calories: | 108 kcal |

Ingredients

2 avocados

1 cup coconut milk

½ cup coconut cream

½ cup cocoa powder

⅓ cup confectioners' sweetener

Optional: drop of vanilla extract

This is how you make the recipe

1. Mix all ingredients together until smooth.

2. Pour mixture into an ice maker and churn for 30 minutes.

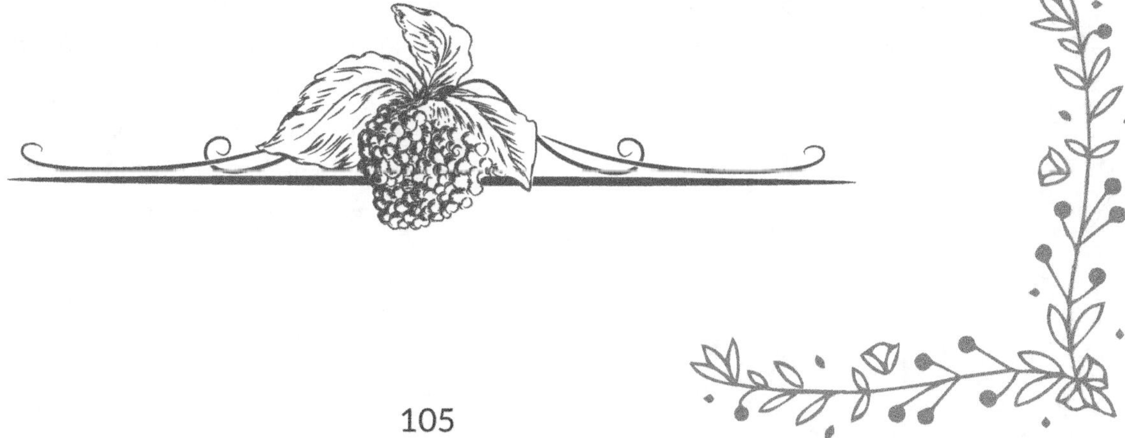

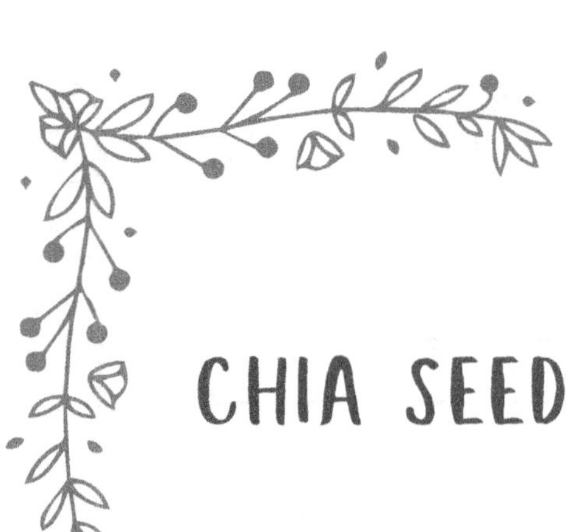

CHIA SEED PUDDING

Ingredients

½ cup heavy cream

1 cup coconut milk

3 tbsp sweetener

2 tsp vanilla extract

⅓ cup chia seeds

This is how you make the recipe

1. Mix all ingredients in a medium bowl until well blended.

2. Let sit for a few minutes and then stir it again.

3. Cover and place in the refrigerator until thick like pudding.

CHOCOLATE PEANUT BUTTER PECAN BARK

Ingredients

1 cup coconut oil

¼ cup cocoa powder

½ cup peanut butter

½ cup sweetener

½ cup shredded coconut

This is how you make the recipe

1. Melt the coconut oil and peanut butter. Stir until creamy.

2. Add the sweetener, coconut and cocoa powder while mixing. Add a pinch of salt to taste.

3. Tip: You can add a teaspoon of vanilla extract for more flavour.

4. Line a baking tray with greaseproof paper. Pour the mixture on the sheet and freeze it for 45 minutes.

5. Remove from the freezer and break into pieces.

CHOCOLATE TOFU PUDDING

Servings: 6

Nutritional Values Per Serving:
Net Carbs: 3 g   Protein: 51 g
Fat: 9 g   Calories: 270 kcal

Ingredients

2 cups tofu

½ cup cocoa powder

2 tbsp sweetener

½ tsp vanilla extract

This is how you make the recipe

1. Mix all ingredients until smooth.

2. Enjoy!

COCONUT COOKIES

Servings: 40

Nutritional Values Per Serving:
Net Carbs: 0 g   Protein: 1 g
Fat: 4 g   Calories: 40 kcal

Ingredients

3 cups shredded coconut

1 cup almond flour

¾ cup sweetener

¼ cup coconut milk

1 cup baking chocolate chips

This is how you make the recipe

1. Line a baking tray with parchment paper.

2. In a bowl, combine all of the ingredients until fully incorporated.

3. Form into small balls and press each ball into a cookie shape.

4. Freeze until firm and enjoy!

MATCHA CUPCAKES

Ingredients

½ cup coconut manna

¼ cup sweetener

½ tsp matcha tea powder

1 tsp baking powder

¼ cup coconut flour

This is how you make the recipe

1. Preheat the oven to 350˚F.

2. Line 6 cups of a muffin tin with cupcake paper

3. Boil ½ cup of water and pour it over the coconut manna. Stir until smooth and combined.

4. Mix in sweetener, matcha tea powder and pinch of salt.

5. Slowly mix in the baking powder and coconut flour until all is well-combined.

6. Put the mixture into the muffin tins and bake for 20 minutes, until the tops are firm.

7. Remove from the oven and allow it to cool.

CREAM CHEESE COOKIES

Ingredients

¼ cup butter, softened

¼ cup soft white cheese (cream cheese)

½ cup sweetener

1 egg white

3 cups almond flour

This is how you make the recipe

1. Preheat the oven to 350˚F. Line a cookie sheet with parchment paper.

2. Beat together the butter and cream cheese until it's fluffy.

3. Add the egg white and a pinch of salt.

4. Beat in the almond flour.

5. Scoop balls of the dough onto the prepared baking tray. Flatten them into biscuits.

6. Bake for 15 minutes.

7. Let them fully cool in the pan until they harden and enjoy!

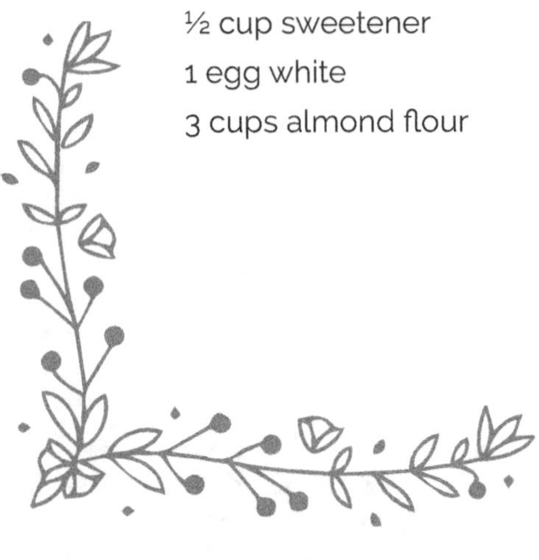

CLOUD CAKE

Servings: 4

Nutritional Values Per Serving:
Net Carbs: 0.8 g — Protein: 5 g
Fat: 12.3 g — Calories: 132 kcal

Ingredients

2 eggs
¼ cup mascarpone cheese
1 tbsp sweetener
Pinch of cream of tartar
¼ tsp instant espresso powder

This is how you make the recipe

1. Preheat the oven to 300°F. Line a baking tray with greaseproof paper.

2. Separate the eggs.

3. Blend together the yolks, mascarpone cheese, sweetener, espresso powder and a pinch of salt.

4. Sprinkle cream of tartar or baking powder on the egg whites and whip until very stiff.

5. Fold the egg yolk mixture into the egg white mixture.

6. Spoon 4 piles of the mixture onto the prepared baking tray and bake for 25-30 minutes.

7. Let them cool before serving.

PUDDING

Servings: 4

Nutritional Values Per Serving:
Net Carbs: 0.7 g — Protein: 12.3 g
Fat: 24.3 g — Calories: 268 kcal

Ingredients

½ cup mascarpone cheese
¼ cup butter
4 eggs, separated
½ tsp sweetener
¼ tsp cream of tartar

This is how you make the recipe

1. In saucepan, melt together the mascarpone cheese and the butter.

2. Mix in the egg yolks and the sweetener.

3. Continue to cook on low heat, stirring occasionally until egg yolks thickens. Then remove from the heat.

4. Sprinkle cream of tartar on the egg whites and whip until very stiff.

5. Beat the egg yolk mixture into the egg whites.

6. Tips: For a more pudding-like consistency, add a tsp of xanthan gum. For taste varieties, you can add lemon zest or vanilla extract or dry raspberries.

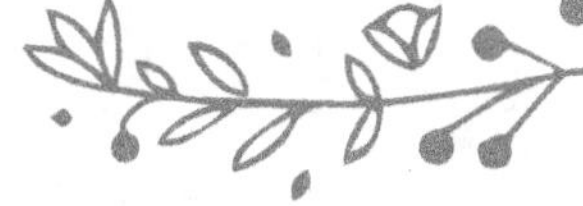

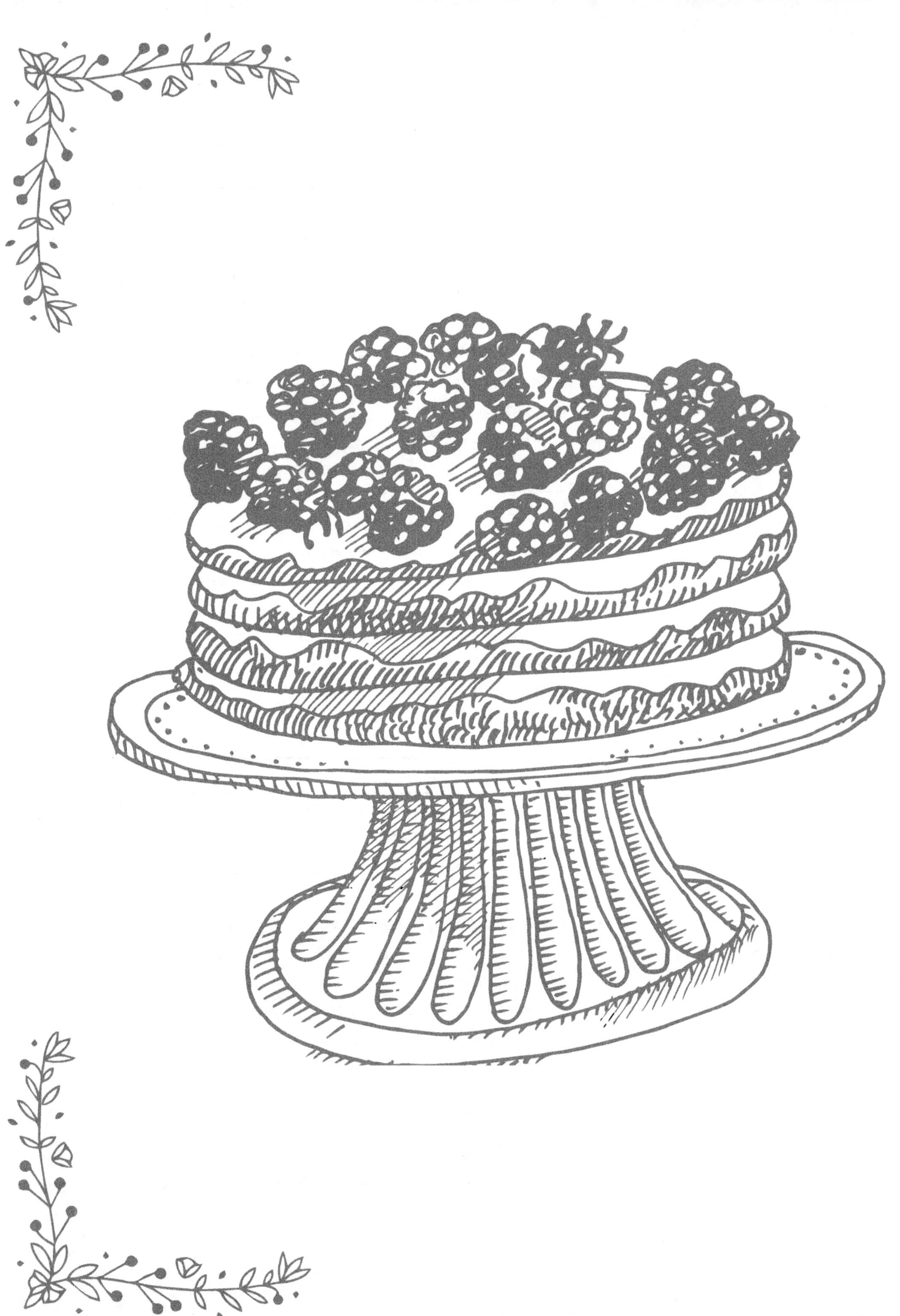

CHOCOLATE CAKE

Ingredients

⅓ cup water

½ cup sweetener

¾ cup baking chocolate chips

⅔ cup butter

4 eggs

This is how you make the recipe

1. Heat the oven to 350°F. Line a spring-form with parchment paper.

2. Melt the chocolate chips and butter together in a double boiler.

3. Add the sweetener and a pinch of salt.

4. One by one, combine the eggs into the chocolate mixture. Beat the mixture well after each egg is added.

5. Pour the mixture into the spring-form and cover with foil.

6. Place the spring-form in a larger pan and add an inch of boiling water to the outside pan.

7. Bake for 45 minutes. Remove and let cool down before removing it from the form.

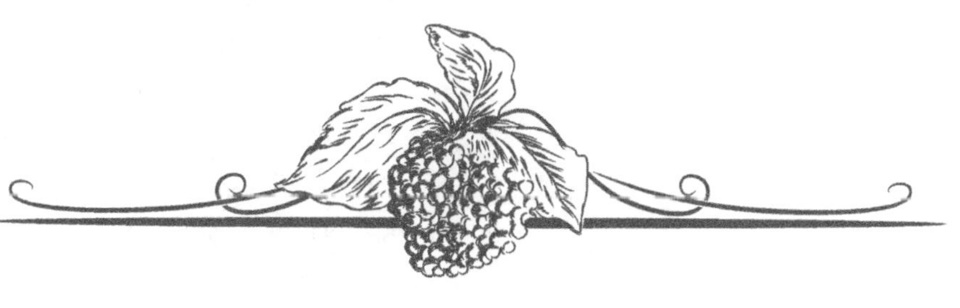

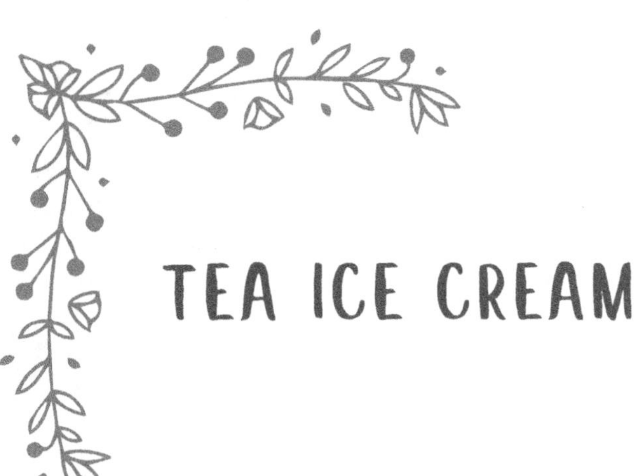

TEA ICE CREAM

Ingredients

⅓ cup boiling water

2 tbsp loose green tea

¼ cup sweetener

½ cup almond milk

1½ cups heavy cream

This is how you make the recipe

1. Boil the tea in a cup of water for 3 minutes.

2. Remove the tea leaves from the water, add sweetener and set aside to cool.

3. Stir in the milk and cream.

4. Pour into an ice cream maker and churn for 20-30 minutes.

5. Serve immediately.

LEMON STRAWBERRY CHEESECAKE JARS

Ingredients

⅓ cup cream cheese, softened

¾ cup heavy cream

⅓ cup sweetener

Zest of 1 lemon

3 strawberries

This is how you make the recipe

1. In a mixing bowl, add the cream cheese, lemon zest, cream and sweetener. Mix until smooth.

2. Chop 2 strawberries into little pieces.

3. Take two jars for serving, use half of the cream cheese mixture to fill up each jar halfway. Reserve the other half of the mixture for the final layer.

4. Add the chopped strawberries to the jars to make a nice central layer.

5. Top the strawberries with the rest of the cream cheese mixture.

6. Then lay on slices of strawberry.

7. Sprinkle lemon zest on the very top and enjoy!

PEANUT BUTTER COOKIE

Servings: 6

Nutritional Values Per Serving:
Net Carbs: 2.5 g Protein: 3 g
Fat: 6 g Calories: 82 kcal

Ingredients

½ cup peanut butter

½ cup powdered sweetener

1 egg

This is how you make the recipe

Preheat oven to 350F. Line a baking tray with greaseproof paper.

In a bowl, put in all the ingredients and mix until well-combined.

Scoop out portions of dough, form balls and place them on the baking tray.

Bake for 12-15 minutes.

Let the biscuits cool before serving.

PEANUT BUTTER FUDGE

Servings: 36

Nutritional Values Per Serving:
Net Carbs: 1 g Protein: 2 g
Fat: 11 g Calories: 109 kcal

Ingredients

1 cup cream cheese

1 cup butter

1 cup peanut butter

1 cup sweetener

½ cup whey protein

This is how you make the recipe

1. In saucepan, melt the cream cheese and butter.

2. Add the peanut butter and stir until well-combined.

3. Remove from heat and mix in the sweetener and whey protein.

4. Pour the mix into a baking dish lined with greaseproof paper.

5. Place in the fridge and let cool.

6. Cut into pieces and enjoy!

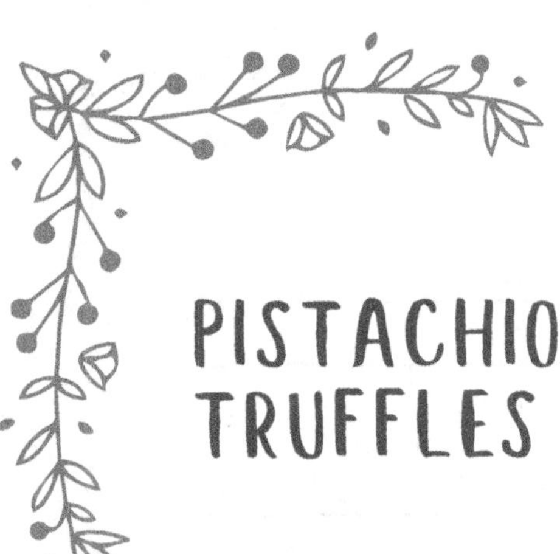

PISTACHIO TRUFFLES

Ingredients

1 cup mascarpone cheese, softened

¼ tsp pure vanilla extract

3 tbsp sweetener

¼ cup pistachios

This is how you make the recipe

1. In a bowl, combine the mascarpone, vanilla and sweetener and mix until smooth.

2. By hand, roll into 10 balls. If it is too soft, refrigerate shortly.

3. Place the chopped pistachios on a plate and coat the truffles.

4. Let them chill before serving and enjoy!

PUMPKIN CUSTARD

Ingredients

1 tin pumpkin puree

1 tsp sweetener

1 tsp cinnamon

4 large egg yolks

¾ cup coconut cream, liquefied

This is how you make the recipe

1. Preheat the oven to 350°F.

2. Combine pumpkin, sweetener and cinnamon in a large bowl. If you wish, mix in ¼ tsp ginger and ⅛ tsp cloves for enhanced flavour.

3. Beat in the egg yolks until incorporated.

4. Slowly stir in the coconut cream.

5. Pour mixture into six ramekins.

6. Bake for 30-40 minutes or until set.

7. Allow to cool on a wire rack.

8. Store in the refrigerator.

STRAWBERRY CHEESECAKES

Servings: 4

Nutritional Values Per Serving:
Net Carbs: 7 g   Protein: 5 g
Fat: 34 g   Calories: 363 kcal

Ingredients

1 cup cream cheese

½ cup heavy cream

2 tbsp sweetener

1 cup strawberries, chopped

¼ cup almond flour

This is how you make the recipe

1. Place the cream cheese and half of the cream into mixer. Mix slowly until combined.

2. Add the remaining cream and the sweetener. Mix again.

3. Add the strawberries and almond flour and stir by hand until well mixed.

4. Spoon into serving dishes.

5. Tip: You can dust a little crushed, freeze-dried strawberry powder on top for a nice taste and decoration if you like.

SHORTBREAD COOKIES

Servings: 24

Nutritional Values Per Serving:
Net Carbs: 0 g   Protein: 2 g
Fat: 6 g   Calories: 64 kcal

Ingredients

¼ cup butter, softened

⅓ cup sweetener

½ tsp vanilla extract

1⅔ cups almond flour

This is how you make the recipe

1. Preheat the oven to 350°F.

2. Mix the butter and sweetener with a hand mixer.

3. Add the vanilla and a pinch of salt.

4. Beat in the almond flour, bit by bit as you mix.

5. Scoop portions of the dough onto a parchment-lined baking sheet and flatten them gently to shape.

6. Bake for 12 minutes, until golden brown at the edges.

7. Allow to cool completely before serving.

RECOMMENDATIONS FOR IDEAL INGREDIENTS

1. For your molds, get one or more molds or mini muffin pans of different sizes. Molds come with as few as 6 cups and as many as 24.
2. Try to use organic ingredients.
3. Grass-fed/pasture-raised dairy products.
4. Himalayan or sea salt.
5. Spring or filtered water.
6. Fresh herbs.
7. Wash your greens and vegetables before cooking.
8. Use baking chocolate which is 100% dark chocolate or use Lily's Stevia sweetened dark chocolate.
9. Sweeteners: Monk fruit is the best for the confections and chocolates. Though Swerve, erythritol, stevia and xylitol are all good sweeteners. Never use synthetic sweeteners
10. Confectioners' sweeteners: Powdered monk fruit, confectioners'Swerve, or powder your own erythritol or xylitol in a coffee grinder
11. Use sugar-free or unsweetened ingredients if not otherwise specified.
12. Coconut milk in a tin rather than powdered coconut milk. Also make sure to use the full-fat type.
13. Cooking oil ; Avocado oil - it has the highest smoke point.